Pathology in
Clinical Practice:
50 Case Studies

Pathology in
Clinical Practice:
50 Case Studies

Barry AT Newell BSc MBBS MRCP FRCPath, Consultant Histopathologist, Department of Cellular
Pathology, St George's Hospital, London, UK

Susan A Dilly BSc MBBS FRCPath, Professor and Institute Director, Institute of Health Sciences
Education, Barts and The London, Queen Mary's School of Medicine and Dentistry, London, UK

Caroline J Finlayson MBBS FRCPath, Honorary Senior Lecturer and Consultant in Histopathology,
St George's Hospital Medical School, London, UK

Mitesh Gandhi MBBS MRCP FRCR FRANZCR, Consultant Radiologist, The Princess Alexandra
Hospital and Queensland X-Ray, Brisbane, Australia

Sunil R Lakhani BSc MBBS MD FRCPath FRCPA, Professor and Head, Molecular and Cellular
Pathology, School of Medicine, University of Queensland, Mayne Medical School, Brisbane, Australia

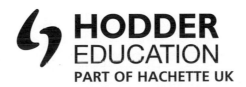
HODDER
EDUCATION
PART OF HACHETTE UK

First published in Great Britain in 2009 by
Hodder Arnold, an imprint of Hodder Education,
part of Hachette UK, 338 Euston Road, London NW1 3BH

http://www.hoddereducation.com

British Library Cataloguing in Publication Data
A catalogue record for this book is available from the British Library

Library of Congress Cataloging-in-Publication Data
A catalog record for this book is available from the Library of Congress

ISBN   978 0 340 95004 6

1 2 3 4 5 6 7 8 9 10

Commissioning Editor: Sara Purdy
Production Editor: Jane Tod and Eva Senior
Production Controller: Karen Dyer
Cover Designer: Helen Townson
Indexer: Dr Laurence Errington

Typeset in 10.5pt Perpetua by Macmillan Publishing Solutions
Printed and bound in Italy

What do you think about this book? Or any other Hodder Arnold title?
Please visit our website: www.hoddereducation.com

This book is dedicated to our families.

CONTENTS

🔎 Sarah McKenzie cases

Nine cases have been written to follow the adventures of a medical student called Sarah McKenzie from her early clinical experience through to her final examinations. These cases create the atmosphere of a clinic, intensive care unit or pathology department and cover some of the topics that students most commonly find difficult, in a way that you should find immediately applicable on your attachment. Several of these cases are a dialogue between Sarah and her clinical teacher designed to encourage clinical reasoning and an appreciation of key concepts. For those students with little clinical experience, it can provide an idea of how best to benefit from apprenticeship-style learning and the potential stress of learning about diseases at the same time as caring for the people suffering from them. Finally, Sarah struggles through a horrendous examination, which should provide encouragement and tactical advice to all students.

PREFACE

In medicine it is always necessary to start with the observation of the sick and to always return to this as this is the paramount means of verification. Observe methodically and vigorously without neglecting any exploratory procedure using all that can be provided by physical examination, chemical studies, bacteriological findings and experiment, one must compare the facts observed during life and the lesions revealed by autopsy.
Antoine Marfan, French paediatrician (1858–1942)

In the last two centuries, medical knowledge has advanced at an amazing rate as bioscientists and clinicians have observed and investigated their patients' conditions to understand better the fundamental mechanisms of disease. That in turn has led to new treatments and the need both to evaluate the effectiveness of the treatment and to identify any detrimental consequences. *Pathology in Clinical Practice* attempts to bring together, in a discussion of 50 scenarios, the basic mechanisms of disease and how they operate to produce the clinical signs and symptoms, a rational approach to investigation and how patient management is influenced by specific pathological phenomena.

This is a companion volume to *Basic Pathology – An introduction to the mechanisms of disease*, which approaches pathology from a clinical perspective, starting with a patient scenario and then working through the detail to cover the molecular and cellular responses to the various disease agents. *Pathology in Clinical Practice* helps students to assess their knowledge of basic pathology and their ability to apply it to their clinical work by using a question-and-answer format. The scenarios increase in complexity through the book, but they can be read in any order. They are broadly arranged into sections familiar to all clinicians as the way in which they approach the patient – first take the history, then elicit the signs, consider the differential diagnosis, assess the need for further investigations and decide on the management. At each of these steps, an appreciation of the fundamental pathological concepts makes clinical medicine both easier to understand and more interesting.

The book uses diagrams to review the mechanisms, colour photographs to illustrate the changes occurring at tissue level and a large number of radiological images that visualize the processes in living patients. The quality, diversity and clinical usefulness of modern imaging allow radiographs to replace what previously might have been available only as a pickled specimen in a pathology museum. Pathology is very much a living subject when studied in this way.

In addition, students will want to learn enough histopathology to be able to interpret a surgical pathology, fine needle aspirate or autopsy report and to explain its significance to their patients. They will enjoy multidisciplinary meetings and clinicopathological conferences much more if the language and images are familiar to them. They will also need to know how to complete a death certificate and when to refer to the coroner. All of this is pathology in clinical practice and is covered in this book.

This book is primarily intended for undergraduate medical students, especially those used to a problem-based learning approach where the pathology is integrated with other subjects. It is written to be accessible to a wide range of students in health and bioscience disciplines and is intended to make revision a stimulating activity that helps join things together in a useful way. The style of some of the scenarios has been varied to provoke reflection on the complexity of clinical practice, including the intricacies of the doctor–patient and student–teacher relationships. Most of all, we hope that this book will encourage students to see pathology as both fun and fundamental.

Barry AT Newell

Susan A Dilly

Caroline J Finlayson

Mitesh Gandhi

Sunil R Lakhani

ACKNOWLEDGEMENT

Healthcare is a collaborative venture with a host of different professionals contributing to patient care and the same is increasingly true of medical education. This book would not have been possible without the help of colleagues who provided advice or illustrations. In particular, we are indebted to people who contributed radiological cases, including Dr Kerry McMahon, Dr Nick Daunt, Dr John Fenwick, Dr Dennis Gribbin, Dr James Fitzgerald, Dr Kendall Redmond, Dr John Andersen, Dr Peter Jackson, Dr Nivene Saad, Dr Thomas Lloyd, Dr Liz Carter, Annette Brennan-Sela, Dominic Kennedy, Kate Lehman, Troy Dobell-Weakley, Dr Murray Thorn, Dr Mohammed Seedat, Dr Phillip Dubois and Dr Piyoosh Kotecha, and a special thanks to Mr Ken Manthey for his invaluable technical advice. Carol Shiels and staff at St George's Pathology Department assisted with many of the macroscopic images. Ann Childs supplied the clinical pictures of Marfan syndrome (Figures 27.2 and 27.3) and Jo Sheldon the M-band illustrations (Figure 23.4). Table 22.1 on vitamin deficiencies is adapted from Lydyard *et al.* (2000) *Pathology Integrated: An A–Z of disease and its pathogenesis*. London: Arnold. We thank Brenda Mason for administrative assistance.

At a more personal level, we are all aware of the time taken away from family and friends when writing a new book and would like to thank our families for their tolerance and support namely: Barry Newell's parents; Mya and Simon Dilly; Rob, Ian and Emma Finlayson; Rohit, Usha, Alka, Milan and Meera Gandhi; Neesha, Meera and Ravi Lakhani.

PART I

SYMPTOMS

A 61-year-old man is referred to the outpatient department at his local hospital with a two-month history of episodic chest pain. The pain is central and radiates to the patient's neck and sometimes to his left arm. The pain is brought on by moderate exertion, such as running up stairs or running for a bus and subsides spontaneously after a few minutes of rest. There are no associated symptoms and the patient has previously been fit and well. Examination is normal.

Question 1

What is the likely diagnosis?

Answer 1

Angina. (Technically the full term is angina pectoris. The word angina simply means tightness or constriction and there are rare, non-cardiac conditions that also use this label, such as Ludwig's angina. However, angina without further qualification is now synonymous with angina pectoris.)

The location of the pain, its radiation, the precipitation by exertion and resolution with rest after just a few minutes are characteristic.

Question 2

What is the cause of the pain in angina?

Answer 2

Angina is the result of myocardial ischaemia. The myocardial ischaemia occurs when blood flow to the affected myocardium is insufficient to meet its metabolic requirements. Given that myocardial metabolism is increased during exertion, this explains the relationship between exertion and precipitation of the pain and why the pain subsides on rest and is absent if this level of exertion is not reached.

Question 3

What is usually the cause of the ischaemia?

Answer 3

The myocardial ischaemia in angina is normally the result of atherosclerosis of one or more coronary arteries. (Prinzmetal angina due to coronary artery vasospasm is uncommon, tends to affect women and occurs at rest.)

Question 4

What are the risk factors for atherosclerosis?

Answer 4

Atherosclerosis is a complex disorder, but there are several important risk factors including:

- smoking
- hypercholesterolaemia
- diabetes mellitus
- hypertension
- family history of atherosclerosis
- male gender.

Question 5

What changes occur to the blood vessel wall in atherosclerosis?

Answer 5

As indicated above, the pathogenesis of atherosclerosis is complex, but the basic process can be summarized as follows.

Atherosclerosis represents a response of a blood vessel to a particular type of injury. Initially, there is damage to the endothelium. This permits the entry of plasma, specifically low-density lipoproteins that transport cholesterol, into the tunica intima of the artery. The aberrantly placed insudated material initiates an inflammatory response in which macrophages are a key component. They ingest the cholesterol and acquire a

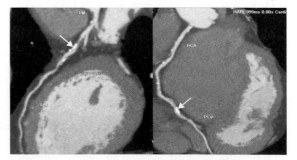

Figure 1.1 CT coronary angiography is used as a non-invasive technique of imaging coronary arteries. These images show multifocal arterial stenoses (arrows), using an intravenous injection of iodinated contrast and a spiral CT scanner. LM, left main artery; LAD, left anterior descending artery; RCA, right coronary artery; PLV, posterior left ventricular artery.

foamy appearance. This fatty element to an atherosclerotic lesion imparts a yellow appearance.

The response is not limited to simply the ingestion of the cholesterol. There is also a fibroblastic proliferation with the production of fibrous tissue. The inflammatory process also recruits the smooth muscle cells of the tunica media, which proliferate and secrete collagen, adding to the atherosclerotic lesion. Very small and fragile new blood vessels may be found at the edges of some atherosclerotic lesions.

The resulting lesion, known as a plaque, comprises a lipid core surrounded by foamy macrophages and fibrous tissue, covered on the luminal aspect by endothelium and associated with a thickened tunica media. Disruption of the internal elastic lamina may also be encountered. Calcification can occur. The plaque occupies a greater volume than the undamaged tunica intima and therefore narrows the lumen of the vessel.

Question 6

How does this produce angina?

Answer 6

In stable angina, the ischaemia is related to a simple mass effect. The atherosclerotic plaque occupies space and narrows the lumen of the blood vessel, thereby reducing the maximum possible blood flow.

Question 7

What complications can occur?

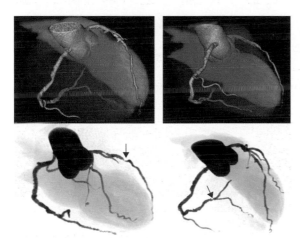

Figure 1.2 Post-processing software allows acquired CT data to be reconstructed producing angiogram-like images. Note the calcified plaque producing stenoses (arrows).

Answer 7

The two main pathological complications are thrombotic and embolic phenomena.

The atherosclerotic plaque is susceptible to further injury. The endothelium overlying the plaque is more fragile than normal and can be sheared off. Damage to the endothelium is one of the triggers for the coagulation cascade and for platelet activation and, if the extent of endothelial injury is sufficient or the degree of pre-existing luminal narrowing caused by the plaque is enough, the resulting thrombus can occlude the lumen of the artery completely. The tissue downstream from the artery will undergo infarction unless it has an adequate collateral blood supply.

Occlusion of the artery can also develop if there is haemorrhage into the plaque, which causes the plaque to expand suddenly and considerably.

Shearing and haemorrhage can also cause part of the plaque to break off and become an embolus which impacts downstream and occludes a distant artery, again leading to organ infarction.

The clinical effect depends on the vessels affected. Hence, the brain may show transient ischaemic attacks and thromboembolic cerebrovascular accidents, the heart can be affected by angina, unstable angina and myocardial infarction, the lower limb may develop intermittent claudication and infarction (peripheral vascular

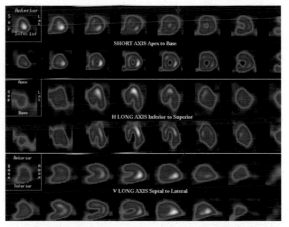

Figure 1.3 Stress/myocardial perfusion test involves injecting intravenous technetium-99m sestamibi followed by maximal exercise on a treadmill or pharmacological stress. The darker areas (arrows) show myocardial underperfusion. This patient demonstrates restoration of perfusion at rest in the ischaemic anterior wall of the heart. Top row in each projection shows stress images; bottom row shows images after 2–4 hours' rest.

The atheromatous plaque

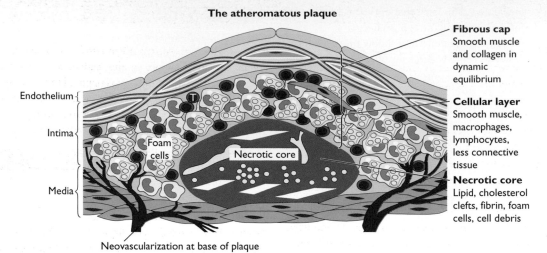

Fibrous cap Smooth muscle and collagen in dynamic equilibrium

Cellular layer Smooth muscle, macrophages, lymphocytes, less connective tissue

Necrotic core Lipid, cholesterol clefts, fibrin, foam cells, cell debris

Endothelium

Intima

Media

Foam cells

Necrotic core

Neovascularization at base of plaque

Figure 1.4 The key components of the atheromatous plaque.

disease), and the gut can exhibit ischaemia or infarction. Furthermore, the damage to the wall of the blood vessel that is caused by atherosclerosis can weaken the wall and yield an aneurysm.

Question 8

How do the risk factors relate to the process of atherogenesis?

Answer 8

Smoking, hypertension and diabetes mellitus can cause endothelial damage.

Hypercholesterolaemia provides an elevated blood level of cholesterol so that any endothelial leakiness will result in more intimal cholesterol than in normal people; diabetes mellitus can also derange lipid metabolism.

A family history of atherosclerotic illness suggests a genetic susceptibility to the generation of atherosclerotic plaques.

Premenopausal levels of oestrogen are believed to have a protective effect against atherosclerosis and this protection is not present in males.

Question 9

What is unstable angina?

Answer 9

Unstable angina is angina that occurs at rest, or on minimal exertion, and loses some of the predictability of stable angina. It is usually associated with a very large and/or unstable atherosclerotic plaque that produces severe narrowing of a coronary artery. This plaque compromises blood flow to such an extent that myocardial perfusion is susceptible to even minor alterations in blood flow such as could occur on trivial exertion.

Question 10

What would the ECG show between attacks in a patient with uncomplicated, stable angina?

Answer 10

Unless there is co-existing hypertensive myocardial damage or another underlying cardiac condition, the ECG would be expected to be normal.

A 23-year-old woman goes to see her GP because she has had several episodes of shortness of breath in the past two months. The episodes last for up to 30 minutes and are sometimes associated with wheezing. She thinks that there is a connection with being exposed to dust as she had her worst episode when she was helping to clean a friend's loft and another episode when she was changing the bag on her vacuum cleaner. She also thinks that cats trigger her shortness of breath. In addition, she has noticed that she sometimes has a dry cough, particularly at night. She has not had a productive cough, haemoptysis or chest pain. She is otherwise fit and well, takes regular exercise and her exercise tolerance remains unchanged.

Question 1

What other questions should form part of a respiratory history?

Answer 1

There are certain items that have a particular significance in the history of a possible respiratory problem. Some of these are specific to a respiratory presentation, while others form part of the more general history. They include the following:

- smoking (type, how many per day, age started, age stopped or if still smoking)
- occupation (occupational dusts and other agents)
- pets or contacts with animals
- hobbies, especially with regard to those involving animals, dusts or chemicals
- asbestos exposure (must inquire specifically)
- history of allergies (patient and relatives)
- history of eczema (patient and relatives)
- history of hay fever (patient and relatives)
- exposure to tuberculosis
- travel abroad
- place of residence.

Question 2

What is the likely diagnosis in this patient's case?

Answer 2

Asthma. The presentation in a young person of episodic dyspnoea that is associated with wheezing and a dry cough and is related to precipitating factors is very suggestive.

Extrinsic allergic alveolitis might also be considered, but the precipitating factors in this patient are somewhat diverse (assorted dusts and cats as opposed to a more specific, single trigger in extrinsic allergic alveolitis) and the cough is not associated with the exposure. The nocturnal exacerbation of the cough is also suggestive of asthma.

Question 3

What is asthma?

Answer 3

Asthma is a chronic condition in which there is bronchial hypersensitivity and hyper-reactivity leading to reversible episodes of bronchospasm that produce dyspnoea and/or wheezing.

Question 4

What is the underlying pathological process?

Answer 4

Asthma is a form of type 1 hypersensitivity reaction. The key components of this response are IgE and mast cells.

The beneficial function of the IgE and mast cell system is in fighting infection by large, parasitic organisms that cannot physically be phagocytosed. Instead, the parasites are bombarded with the contents of the toxic granules that are released from mast cells. These contents include histamine, which has a bronchoconstrictor action.

The generation of a co-ordinated and targeted mast cell response against an infection can be mediated by IgE. The IgE molecules bind to the parasite. Mast cells bear specific receptors for IgE on their cell membrane. Binding of multiple IgE antibodies to the receptors on a mast cell activates the mast cell and triggers the release of its granules. In this way, the potentially harmful and destructive substances within the granules are focused against the microorganism and are not released into the tissues without good cause. However, in asthma, this process is disrupted and behaves in an aberrant and harmful fashion.

Many of the inhaled agents that precipitate asthma share the property of possessing a repeated antigenic sequence that is recognized by an IgE antibody. Therefore, if the patient has IgE antibodies that are specific for that sequence, exposure to the precipitant will result in the binding of numerous IgE molecules to it. This array of IgE molecules closely arranged on the precipitant is a potent stimulator of mast cells, leading to an exaggerated response, or type 1 hypersensitivity reaction.

Many different inhaled substances can trigger asthma. The faeces of the house dust mite are among the most common precipitants, but pollen and animal hair and fur are also frequent. In some patients, the trigger may be more difficult to relate directly to activation of the mast cell system, such as exercise or stress.

While histamine produces the acute features that are seen in asthma within an hour of exposure to the trigger, a second reaction can follow around 8–12 hours later and is caused by the production of arachidonic acid metabolites. Unlike the release of histamine by the mast cells, the generation of prostaglandins and leukotrienes requires this period of 8–12 hours to exert an effect. Eosinophils become recruited in this later response and, like mast cells, have a role in the response to parasites, again by the release of toxic granules.

Question 5

How does the underlying pathology explain the symptoms?

Answer 5

The substances released by mast cells are bronchoconstrictors. Narrowing of the airways impairs movement of air in and out of the lungs, producing dyspnoea. Sufficient narrowing will also generate wheeze. Mucus production is also stimulated by the immune response in asthma and this excess mucus exacerbates the effects of the bronchoconstriction.

The inhaled nature of many of the precipitants (dust, animal hair) accounts for the lung-specific manifestation of the hypersensitivity reaction. The antigen is delivered to the lungs and elicits the response there. This principle also applies to extrinsic allergic alveolitis (although this is a type 3 hypersensitivity reaction).

Between attacks, people with asthma typically have normal lung function, reflecting the fact that, in the absence of exposure to a precipitant, the hypersensitivity response that underlies the disease is dormant and exerts no effect on the lungs. Viewed from the other perspective, the episodic but often stereotyped asthmatic response to exposure to a trigger is caused by the immune reaction being activated by the relevant antigen. Furthermore, once the precipitant is removed, the response subsides and normal function returns.

The danger of an exacerbation of asthma flaring up several hours after the initial attack has resolved is a

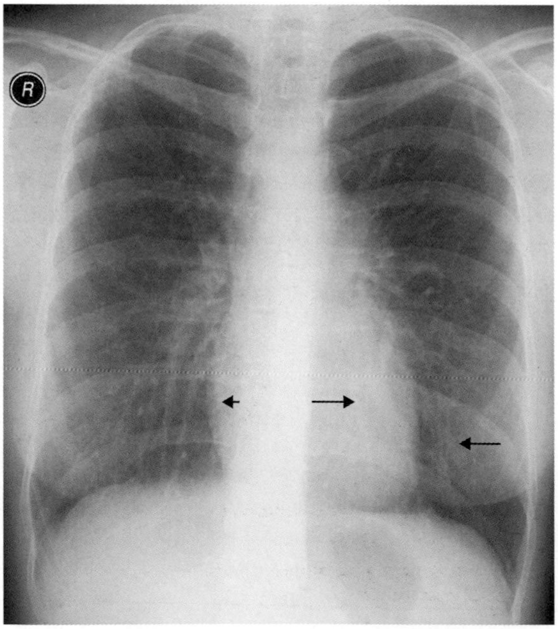

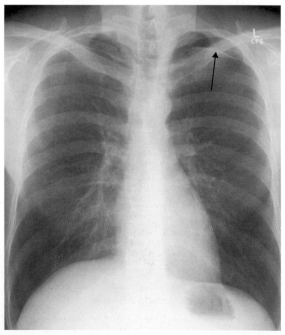

Figure 2.1 Chest X-ray in acute asthma showing overinflated lungs (a consequence of air trapping) together with peribronchial thickening (arrows).

Figure 2.2 Chest X-ray showing an apical pneumothorax in a child with asthma. High intra-alveolar pressures in acute asthma can lead to alveolar rupture with escape of air into the pleural space (a pneumothorax – arrow) and collapse of the underlying lung.

consequence of the slower acting arachidonic acid cascade taking time to recruit other cells to the process.

A characteristic feature of asthma is the tendency for bronchospasm to develop during the early hours of the morning. The cause for this is not clear, but may reflect circadian rhythms in substances such as corticosteroids. However, it is of clinical importance because a patient admitted with a severe exacerbation of asthma should demonstrate a stable condition overnight, while taking only the medications on which he or she is intended to be discharged, before being sent home. Rushing this step can result in the exacerbation flaring up again in the early hours of the morning, which is not the safest time for it to happen.

Question 6

What is anaphylactic shock?

Answer 6

Anaphylatic shock is an extreme form of type 1 hypersensitivity reaction that occurs on a systemic scale. There is widespread release of mast cell contents leading to vasodilatation and hypotension, as well as bronchospasm and airway oedema. The condition can be fatal. Bee stings are one of the better known triggers.

Question 7

What investigations are of value in asthma?

Answer 7

The diagnosis of asthma is essentially clinical. Any investigations are generally to exclude other conditions, but could include the following.

- Full blood count (FBC) (anaemia can exacerbate respiratory problems, elevated white cell count (WCC) may suggest an infective element; mild eosinophilia can be found in allergic conditions)
- Chest X-ray (should be normal; valuable in very young children to exclude a foreign body).

(The investigations required in an acute exacerbation of asthma are not discussed.)

Of considerably more importance for longer term management is measurement of the peak expiratory flow rate (PEFR). This is simple and quick to undertake and can be done by patients themselves at

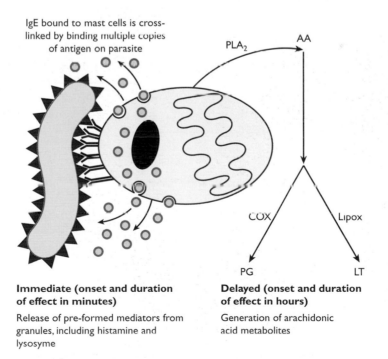

IgE bound to mast cells is cross-linked by binding multiple copies of antigen on parasite

PLA$_2$ AA

COX Lipox

PG LT

Immediate (onset and duration of effect in minutes)

Release of pre-formed mediators from granules, including histamine and lysosyme

Delayed (onset and duration of effect in hours)

Generation of arachidonic acid metabolites

Figure 2.3 Mast cell activation is typically stimulated by IgE antibody cross-linkage as illustrated here, but this is not always necessary. Mast cells can also be directly stimulated by some substances, e.g. mellitin from bee stings or C3a5A complement fragments.

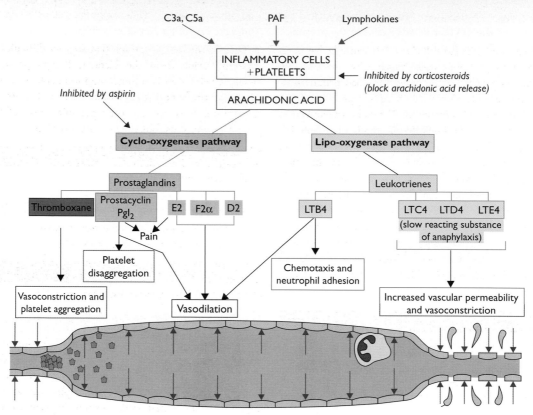

Figure 2.4 Sources and effects of the major cytokines involved in inflammation.

home. Patients should be given a PEFR meter and a chart on which to document their PEFR. The PEFR should be recorded a few times during the day, at the same times each day, for a few weeks after the initial diagnosis. They should also record their PEFR if they feel short of breath or wake up during the night. Establishing a patient's normal PEFR is important as this can provide a baseline for determining the degree of aggressiveness of treatment in any exacerbations of the asthma.

A 72-year-old man consults his GP because he has been troubled by problems passing urine for the last few months. In particular, the patient has had problems in starting to urinate. This is mirrored by a protracted end to each episode of micturition. When he thinks he has finished urinating he finds that he tends to dribble for more than a few seconds and confides that, on a couple of occasions, this has nearly led to embarrassing incidents when he was using public toilets. On being asked by the GP, he indicates that his urinary stream is not as strong as it was when he was younger and that urination takes longer than it used to. Other than the problems with the dribbling, the patient has not had any episodes of urinary incontinence. There have been no alterations in his bowel habit or problems with faecal continence.

Question I

What is the likely diagnosis?

Answer I

Benign prostatic hyperplasia (BPH).

The patient has symptoms that suggest difficulty in expelling urine from the bladder. Benign prostatic hyperplasia is a very common condition in older men in which enlargement of the prostate narrows the prostatic urethra. It is not the only possible cause of the patient's symptoms, but is by far the most likely.

Question 2

What is hyperplasia?

Answer 2

Hyperplasia is an increase in the size of a tissue or organ due an increase in the number of its cells.

Question 3

How is hyperplasia different from hypertrophy?

Answer 3

Hypertrophy is an increase in the size of a tissue or an organ due to an increase in the size of the individual cells of that tissue or organ without an increase in the number of cells. The term 'hypertrophy' can also be applied to individual cells. Often hyperplasia and hypertrophy occur together.

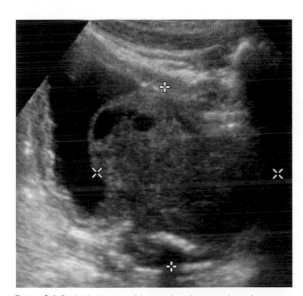

Figure 3.1 Sagittal ultrasound image showing an enlarged prostate indenting the bladder. Ultrasound assesses the kidneys for hydronephrosis and stones. Bladder volumes can be assessed following micturition to determine the degree of post-micturition residual left in the bladder – an assessment of the functional effect of prostatomegaly.

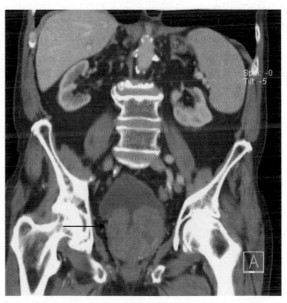

Figure 3.2 Coronal CT showing indentation of the bladder base by an enlarged prostate (arrow).

Question 4

How does prostatic hyperplasia explain the patient's symptoms?

Answer 4

The prostate gland is located immediately inferior to the neck of the bladder and encircles the prostatic urethra. The enlargement of the prostate secondary to the hyperplasia can partially occlude the urethra and many of the symptoms that follow are simply manifestations of obstruction of a pipe that carries fluid from a reservoir.

Hesitancy at the start of micturition reflects difficulties in initiating the flow of urine through the obstructed urethra. The narrowing of the urethra reduces the maximum flow, resulting in a greater time required to empty the bladder, and also increases the resistance to flow, such that the urinary stream emerges at a lower pressure. The phenomenon of terminal dribbling is related to this.

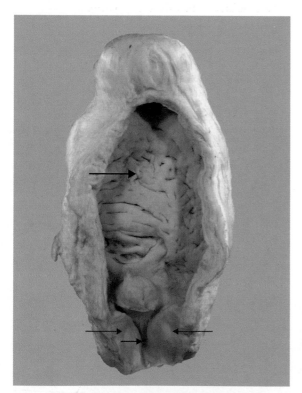

Figure 3.3 The prostate (red arrows) surrounds and compresses the prostatic urethra (black arrow), obstructing urine outflow. The bladder muscle has undergone hypertrophy and the wall shows trabeculation (blue arrow) instead of the normal smooth lining.

Question 5

What secondary changes could occur in the bladder?

Answer 5

Most hollow muscular organs of the body share the same responses to obstruction to their outflow. Hypertrophy of their muscles, either smooth muscle in the case of the bladder and bowel, or cardiac muscle in the heart, is a response that attempts to overcome the obstruction by making the organ capable of generating a greater expulsive/propulsive pressure. This is a consequence of the physiological properties of muscle fibres, which naturally undergo hypertrophy in the face of an increased load.

If the organ cannot expel adequately against the obstruction, the accumulation of its contents will lead to dilatation.

Dilatation and hypertrophy may be found in combination or isolation.

Question 6

What symptoms could result from these changes in the bladder?

Answer 6

As well as the obstructive symptoms of benign prostatic hyperplasia, as experienced by this patient, there can be irritative symptoms. These reflect alterations in the behaviour of the bladder secondary to hypertrophy and/or dilatation. Patients can experience a sense of urinary urgency in which they suddenly develop a strong urge to urinate, even though the volume of urine passed may be small and disproportionate to the magnitude of the urge. Related to this is the symptom of frequency in which the patient needs to urinate more often than

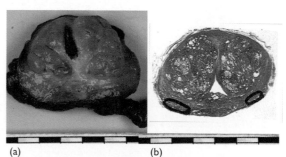

(a)   (b)

Figure 3.4 Transverse slice through prostate with benign prostatic hypertrophy. (a) Fresh specimen. (b) Microscopy, wholemount, with small foci of prostatic carcinoma (indicated) in a characteristically posterior peripheral distribution.

normal, again passing only small volumes. Disruption to the functions of the urinary sphincters can also play a role in both the obstructive and irritative symptoms of BPH.

Nocturia is one of the most troublesome symptoms of BPH because it wakes the patient from sleep on one, a few or multiple occasions during the night.

Question 7

What other phenomena can occur in BPH?

Answer 7

The obstruction in BPH means that incomplete emptying of the bladder can occur, leaving a residual volume of urine. As is typical of the presence of stagnant fluid in other organs of the body (for example, a region of lung distal to an obstructed airway), bacterial super infection can occur. In BPH, this leads to urinary tract infections, which are normally unusual in males.

The blockage to the outflow of urine from the bladder can cause the pressure in the bladder to be transmitted back up the ureter to the renal pelvis, culminating in hydronephrosis and even chronic renal failure.

In some patients, the BPH results in complete occlusion of the urethra. This process may involve elements of infection, oedema and spasm of the urinary sphincters.

The patient is completely unable to pass urine and suffers acute, very painful distension of the bladder that necessitates catheterization.

Question 8

How does BPH differ from prostatic carcinoma?

Answer 8

At the most fundamental level, benign prostatic hyperplasia is a benign process, whereas prostatic carcinoma is a malignant disease. Although both can cause enlargement of the prostate and the associated symptoms, BPH tends to affect the central regions of the prostate while prostatic carcinoma more often commences in the peripheral regions of the gland. This implies that BPH has a greater tendency to cause obstructive symptoms and at an earlier stage.

In BPH, the prostate gland retains a smooth surface, except in extreme examples. In prostatic carcinoma the gland is typically asymmetrically enlarged and irregular and can be hard, rather than soft to firm.

Prostate-specific antigen (PSA) is a substance synthesized by the prostate. Its levels may be elevated in both BPH and prostatic carcinoma. However, very high levels tend to be found only in carcinoma, especially in metastatic disease

A 62-year-old man presents to his GP with a three-month history of difficulty in swallowing. This has been accompanied by a reduction in appetite and weight loss of 7 kg. The dysphagia is mainly for solids. Examination is unremarkable.

g. motor neurone disease
h. myasthenia gravis
i. Parkinson's disease
j. myopathy
k. diffuse oesophageal spasm.

Question 1

What are the causes of dysphagia?

Answer 1

The causes of dysphagia can be considered under four categories. The blockage may be caused by something within the lumen or arising from the mucosal lining, a mass within the wall of the tube, a mass that compresses the tube from the outside or a motility disorder that impairs co-ordinated muscular contraction of the tube. Some causes can fit into more than one category. For swallowing this list is quite long, particularly as swallowing involves not only the oesophagus, but also the pharynx and associated structures:

1. Intraluminal/mucosal:
   a. benign oesophageal stricture
   b. oesophageal malignancy
   c. benign neoplasm (e.g. leiomyoma)
   d. Plummer–Vinson syndrome
   e. Schatzki ring
   f. oesophagitis
2. Wall:
   a. pharyngeal pouch
   b. oesophageal malignancy
3. Extrinsic:
   a. goitre
   b. bronchial carcinoma
   c. mediastinal tumour (e.g. lymphoma)
   d. enlarged left atrium
   e. aortic arch aneurysm
   f. aberrant mediastinal vascular anatomy
   g. peritonsillar abscess
   h. pharyngeal pouch
4. Motility:
   a. hiatus hernia
   b. achalasia
   c. Chagas' disease
   d. scleroderma
   e. cerebrovascular accident
   f. multiple sclerosis

Question 2

Can the dysphagia and weight loss be linked?

Answer 2

If the dysphagia is of a sufficient degree to reduce the patient's food intake significantly, then weight loss may arise. However, if the dysphagia is due to a malignant tumour, the weight loss could be a consequence of tumour cachexia, as well as or instead of a reduced food intake.

Question 3

The GP initiates a set of investigations. These include an upper gastrointestinal (GI) endoscopy. A tumour is seen at 28 cm at endoscopy. The biopsy report reveals a moderately differentiated squamous cell carcinoma. What is a carcinoma?

Answer 3

A carcinoma is a malignant tumour derived from epithelium. A malignant tumour is one that has the capacity to invade and metastasize.

Question 4

What is meant by the term 'differentiation' when applied to a tumour?

Answer 4

Differentiation is an assessment of how closely the malignant tumour resembles the tissues from which it arose. For most tumours, a three-tier system is employed, but there are exceptions. A well-differentiated tumour shares many cytological and architectural features with the tissue of origin and exhibits relatively little disorganization. A poorly differentiated tumour bears little resemblance to the tissue of origin. Moderately differentiated tumours fall in between. In colloquial terms, the differentiation of a carcinoma is a measure of how nasty it looks.

The differentiation of a tumour is also referred to as the grade of the tumour.

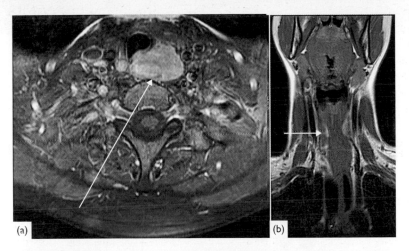

Figure 4.1 (a) A T$_1$-weighted MR study post-intravenous contrast showing a cervical oesophageal cancer (arrowhead) invading the trachea (thin arrow). (b) Coronal T$_1$-weighted MR scan showing a cervical oesophageal squamous cell carcinoma (SCC) (arrow).

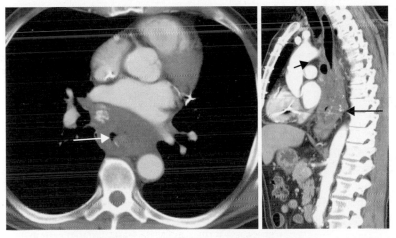

Figure 4.2 Axial and sagittal CT showing a mid-oesophageal cancer producing circumferential thickening of the oesophageal wall and constriction of the lumen (arrows).

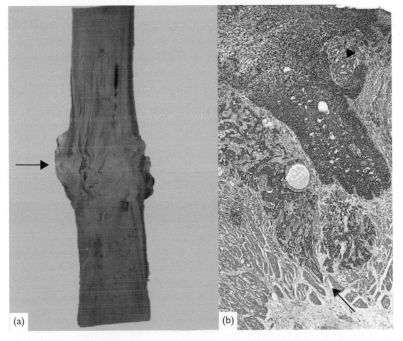

Figure 4.3 (a) Oesophagus opened longitudinally showing an annular tumour present in the middle (arrow). (b) Microscopic appearance of an invasive squamous cell carcinoma of the oesophagus (arrow) arising in squamous mucosa which shows dysplasia (arrowhead) (disordered maturation and cytological atypia).

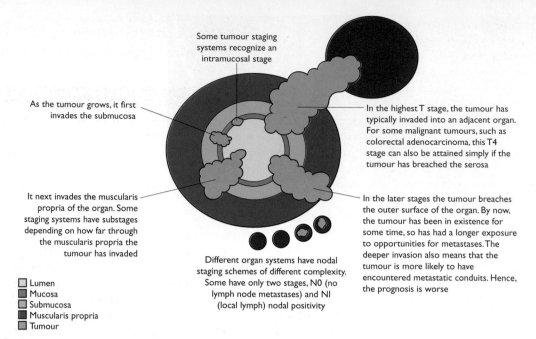

Some tumour staging systems recognize an intramucosal stage

As the tumour grows, it first invades the submucosa

In the highest T stage, the tumour has typically invaded into an adjacent organ. For some malignant tumours, such as colorectal adenocarcinoma, this T4 stage can also be attained simply if the tumour has breached the serosa

It next invades the muscularis propria of the organ. Some staging systems have substages depending on how far through the muscularis propria the tumour has invaded

In the later stages the tumour breaches the outer surface of the organ. By now, the tumour has been in existence for some time, so has had a longer exposure to opportunities for metastases. The deeper invasion also means that the tumour is more likely to have encountered metastatic conduits. Hence, the prognosis is worse

Different organ systems have nodal staging schemes of different complexity. Some have only two stages, N0 (no lymph node metastases) and N1 (local lymph) nodal positivity

☐ Lumen
◼ Mucosa
◼ Submucosa
◼ Muscularis propria
◼ Tumour

Figure 4.4 Schematic cross-section through the oesophagus, illustrating how the TNM system is used to express the stage of tumour spread. T = extent of local tumour spread. N = extent of spread to lymph nodes. M = distant metastatic disease (M0, absent, M1 present).

Almost all carcinomas need to be graded for each individual patient. Other categories of tumour, such as sarcomas, tend to have a grade assigned to the different types by definition. For example, dermatofibrosarcoma protuberans is considered to be a low-grade sarcoma, while synovial sarcoma is a high-grade sarcoma.

Question 5

What is the significance of the grade of a malignant tumour?

Answer 5

Grade has consistently been shown to be a prognostic factor across many types of malignant neoplasm. The higher the grade (and the more poorly differentiated the tumour), the worse the prognosis.

Question 6

The patient undergoes some other investigations, including imaging studies. The oncologist explains to the patient that these are part of the process of staging the carcinoma. What is staging?

Answer 6

The stage of a malignant tumour is a measure of how far the tumour has spread. For carcinomas, this spread is considered relative to the epithelium of the organ of origin.

Tumours of different organs have different staging criteria. These have been determined in particular detail for carcinomas. Common to all carcinomas is the use of the TNM (tumour, node, metastasis) system.

The TNM classification breaks the staging down into three components: the primary tumour, the local lymph nodes and the distant metastases. Each component is assigned a number. For example, a colorectal carcinoma that invades beyond the muscularis propria, but does not breach the serosa and has metastases in two local lymph nodes but no distant metastases, would be staged at T3 N1 M0. Different patterns of the T, N and M parameters can be converted to stages 1–4 if desired.

Some organs have a staging system that operates in parallel to the TNM scheme. The best example is Dukes' staging system for colorectal carcinoma.

Question 7

What is the importance of staging?

Answer 7

Staging is almost always the single most important prognostic factor for any given malignancy. Spread of the tumour beyond its place of origin is the principal mechanism by which a malignant tumour causes morbidity and mortality. In addition, the suitability of surgery as a treatment option is dependent on stage. Low-stage tumours can be very amenable to surgery as resection removes all of the disease. As tumours attain a higher stage, the required surgery becomes more radical and there is a greater danger that the patient already harbours occult distant metastases that are too small to detect with current imaging technology. These distant metastases will not be cleared by the surgery and will continue to grow. For these higher-stage tumours, radiotherapy and/or chemotherapy may afford a better prognosis. (There are exceptions where this situation is paradoxically reversed, or more complex, such as some head and neck tumours.)

Accurate staging of a patient is vital because it can prevent the patient being subjected to radical surgery and/or chemoradiotherapy when there is no real chance of cure and palliative options would have a greater benefit, or conversely when cure could be achieved through less aggressive therapy because the tumour is at an early stage. Conversely, accurate staging is also essential to ensure that a patient receives therapy that is appropriately aggressive in order to maximize the chances of cure if such a possibility exists.

Staging guides treatment to optimize it such that it is neither too mild nor too aggressive. This function is intrinsically linked to the close relationship between stage and prognosis.

Question 8

Which parameter dominates the prognosis, stage or grade?

Answer 8

In almost all tumours, stage trumps grade by a considerable distance.

Question 9

What other prognostic parameters can be assessed on the resected specimen?

Answer 9

Different tumours have their own prognostic nuances. However, many share the parameter of lymphovascular invasion. If the tumour has gained access to the lymphovascular system, it has a route of distant spread away from the primary site. Thus, the presence of lymphovascular invasion frequently indicates a worse prognosis.

Perineural invasion is similar to lymphovascular invasion, but in this case the tumour invades inside the sheath of a nerve and uses the nerve fibre as a highway out of the primary site. Perineural invasion often fails to achieve significance as an independent prognostic indicator for many tumours.

With the growing use of hormonal and other molecular targeted therapies, the expression of specific molecules by the tumour can be of prognostic value. The most frequent example is breast carcinoma in which the expression by the carcinoma of oestrogen receptors is associated with a better prognosis and provides an additional avenue of treatment.

A 25-year-old woman goes to see her GP because she has been troubled for the last two months by a tendency to bruise very easily. During this time, her menstrual periods have also been much heavier than usual. There has not been any haemoptysis, haematemesis, melaena or the passage of fresh blood per rectum. The patient has no other symptoms and has previously been fit and well. She is not taking any medication. Examination is unremarkable.

Question 1

What are the basic elements involved in initiating clotting of the blood?

Answer 1

The initiation of a blood clot is a complex process that is dependent on the properties of the blood flow, the endothelium of the blood vessel and the contents of the blood (Virchow's triad).

Answer 1a

Normal blood flow is smooth and laminar. If blood flow becomes turbulent, this can trigger clotting. Turbulent flow will develop at the site of an injury if the wall of the blood vessel is breached and blood can escape. However, turbulent flow can also arise in blood vessels that are severely narrowed by a pathological process such as atherosclerosis, or in the eddies that may develop in an aneurysm, in both of which cases the resulting clot can be harmful rather than protective.

Answer 1b

While the response to turbulent blood flow can be contributory, additional systems are necessary to ensure that the clotting process is initiated when it is required and the endothelium is central to this. Under normal circumstances, the endothelium provides a smooth lining to the blood vessels and provides a surface that does not encourage clotting. However, if the endothelium is damaged, the underlying tissue is exposed allowing tissue factor, which is a potent trigger for the initiation of clotting, to come into contact with the blood. The inflammatory response that accompanies tissue damage also involves mediators that promote clotting.

The endothelium is not just a passive participant in clotting. Damaged endothelium upregulates procoagulant proteins and also releases vasoconstricting factors. Local vasoconstriction is a protective response which reduces the blood flow into the breach and therefore decreases blood loss.

Answer 1c

The ability of the endothelium and disturbances of blood flow to trigger clotting is effective only if the blood possesses the capacity to clot. This is bestowed by the coagulation cascade and the platelets.

The coagulation cascade consists of a series of proteins, each of which can exist in an inactive and active state. An active protein can activate one or more proteins further down the sequence, the final goal of the

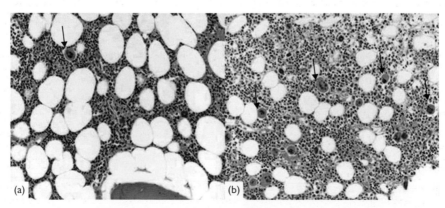

Figure 5.1 (a) Bone marrow that shows a normal number of megakaryocytes relative to the overall cellularity. (b) Bone marrow in idiopathic thrombocytopenic purpura in which there is hyperplasia of the megakaryocytes (arrows).

cascade being to drive the conversion of fibrinogen to fibrin. Fibrin forms a cross-linked network of fibres which spans the breach in the blood vessel and entangles erythrocytes and platelets within it. It forms the scaffold on which the clot is built.

The coagulation cascade is shown in Figure 5.2. The biological relevance of the traditional division into the intrinsic and extrinsic pathways is currently under scrutiny, although it retains some usefulness when considering the meaning of certain tests of blood clotting. Cascades occur in various physiological processes and, while their details can be frustrating to learn, it is important to remember certain basic features that a cascade system confers.

Using a cascade to bring about a final process allows for amplification of a small initial stimulus into a very powerful ultimate response. For example, if a cascade has five steps and one molecule at each stage can activate ten molecules in the next stage, one activated molecule at the top of the cascade could yield up to 10 000 activated end products. In the formation of the blood clot, this amplification is desirable because the breach to the circulation needs to be sealed quickly and effectively.

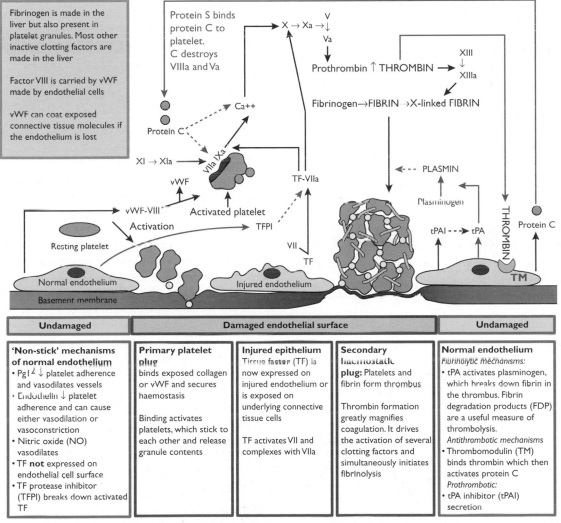

Undamaged	Damaged endothelial surface			Undamaged
'Non-stick' mechanisms of normal endothelium • PgI₂ ↓ platelet adherence and vasodilates vessels • Endothelin ↓ platelet adherence and can cause either vasodilation or vasoconstriction • Nitric oxide (NO) vasodilates • TF **not** expressed on endothelial cell surface • TF protease inhibitor (TFPI) breaks down activated TF	**Primary platelet plug** binds exposed collagen or vWF and secures haemostasis Binding activates platelets, which stick to each other and release granule contents	**Injured epithelium** Tissue factor (TF) is now expressed on injured endothelium or is exposed on underlying connective tissue cells TF activates VII and complexes with VIIa	**Secondary haemostatic plug:** Platelets and fibrin form thrombus Thrombin formation greatly magnifies coagulation. It drives the activation of several clotting factors and simultaneously initiates fibrinolysis	**Normal endothelium** *Fibrinolytic mechanisms:* • tPA activates plasminogen, which breaks down fibrin in the thrombus. Fibrin degradation products (FDP) are a useful measure of thrombolysis. *Antithrombotic mechanisms* • Thrombomodulin (TM) binds thrombin which then activates protein C *Prothrombotic:* • tPA inhibitor (tPAI) secretion

Figure 5.2 Platelet aggregates ('primary platelet plugs') can plug small breaches in the endothelium, but serious tears require the addition of a fibrin mesh (generated by the coagulation cascade) to stabilize the platelets and form thrombus while healing takes place. vWF, von Willebrand factor.

Having multiple elements in a cascade permits more complex modification of the cascade. Different substances outside the cascade can modulate the function of different parts of the cascade. This can afford a greater degree of control and regulation than if the pathway consisted of only a couple of components.

Even a fully formed fibrin scaffold is insufficient to seal a breached blood vessel in the absence of patches to cover it. These patches are provided by the platelets.

Although platelets contain various enzyme systems and granules, possess assorted surface membrane receptors and have microtubule arrays that let them change shape, they lack a nucleus, are much smaller than normal cells and are not classified as cells as such. Instead, they are the fragments of much larger progenitor cells called megakaryocytes which develop in the bone marrow then split into multiple pieces to generate platelets. Platelets become entrapped in the fibrin matrix and are instrumental in forming the blood clot, but their role in the process is not simply that of a passive patch. Platelets are active agents, able to secrete both procoagulant and anticoagulant factors, as well as having adhesive properties that allow them to bind to damaged endothelium and each other, in addition to being able to change shape. Indeed, small breaches in a blood vessel can be sealed by a mass of aggregated platelets without the need to invoke the coagulation cascade.

Question 2

What simple tests are available to assess clotting?

Answer 2

The simplest evaluation of clotting would include a full blood count and the basic clotting profile.

The full blood count includes the platelet count. The platelet count alone does not give any indication of the functional capacity of the platelets, but disorders of platelet function, as opposed to platelet numbers, are rare. Tests of platelet function are available if required.

The basic clotting profile typically provides at least three parameters: the international normalized ratio (INR), activated partial thromboplastin time (ratio) (APTT(R)) and the thrombin time. Each of these focuses on a different part of the coagulation cascade.

The INR is directly derived from the prothrombin time and is the ratio of the patient's prothrombin time to a standard prothrombin time. The INR detects defects in the extrinsic and common parts of the clot-ting cascade and is useful for identifying problems that relate to fibrinogen and factors II, V, VII and X. The main action of the anticoagulant drug warfarin is on these aspects of coagulation and therefore the INR is used to monitor warfarin therapy.

The APTT(R) deals with the intrinsic and common parts of the cascade and discerns problems with fibrinogen and factors II, V, VIII, IX, X and XII. The APTT(R) can be used to monitor the effects of intravenous heparin (now often superseded by low-molecular-weight heparins).

The thrombin time has a more limited range and concentrates on thrombin and fibrinogen.

Fibrinogen levels may also be included in the basic clotting profile.

Question 3

The patient has a normal clotting profile but her full blood count reveals a platelet count of 39; her haemoglobin and white cell count are normal. What descriptive term is given to a low platelet count?

Answer 3

Thrombocytopenia.

Question 4

A diagnosis is suspected and a bone marrow biopsy is undertaken to confirm it. The bone marrow trephine has normal erythropoiesis and myelopoiesis but demonstrates a significant increase in the number of megakaryocytes. Other than the increase in number, the megakaryocytes do not exhibit abnormal features. How can hyperplasia of the megakaryocyte population be related to a decrease in the number of platelets in the peripheral blood?

Answer 4

If the platelet count falls due to some process that destroys or sequesters platelets once they enter the peripheral blood, the appropriate response of the bone marrow would be to increase megakaryopoiesis in order to generate more platelets and return peripheral blood levels to normal. Thus, the changes in this patient's bone marrow are appropriate to her condition.

Question 5

What is the diagnosis (the patient's viral serology is negative)?

Answer 5

The patient has idiopathic thrombocytopenic purpura (ITP). ITP is a common cause of a reduced platelet count, but alternative conditions such as drug-induced thrombocytopenia, virus-related thrombocytopenia and bone marrow failure must be excluded. This process of exclusion is typical of the diagnostic approach in many idiopathic diseases.

Question 6

What is this cause of this condition?

Answer 6

Idiopathic thrombocytopenic purpura is an autoimmune condition in which the patient produces antibodies that are directed against his or her own platelets. Occasionally, the antibodies may operate at the megakaryocyte level and the typical megakaryocyte hyperplasia is not seen in the bone marrow.

A 64-year-old woman presents to her GP with a three-month history of increased breathlessness and occasional episodes of haemoptysis. She is known to have chronic obstructive pulmonary disease (COPD) but thinks that her shortness of breath is worse than she normally expects from her condition. It is also not typical of the infective exacerbations with which she is familiar. She is very worried by the haemoptysis.

Her previous medical history includes COPD and hypertension. Her hypertension is controlled with an ACE inhibitor. She smoked 15 cigarettes per day from the age of 20 to 60 (when her COPD was diagnosed).

Examination of her cardiovascular and abdominal systems is unremarkable. There is a mild reduction in expansion in the right lower zone, the percussion note is a little dull and the breath sounds are quiet relative to elsewhere.

Question 1

What diagnosis must be considered?

Answer 1

In a patient of this age who is a smoker or ex-smoker and presents with haemoptysis, bronchial carcinoma is a definite possibility, particularly in the absence of infection as an alternative cause.

Question 2

The GP arranges an urgent referral to the local chest clinic, but receives a request for a home visit from the patient four days later. Her dyspnoea has worsened and she now has a cough that is productive of green sputum. She has pain on inspiration on the right side of her chest. Examination reveals decreased expansion on the right side of the chest that is of a greater degree than four days previously. The percussion note is dull over the right lower zone, again to a greater degree than when the patient was first examined. The breath sounds over the right lower zone are quiet and have the quality of bronchial breathing. The breath sounds elsewhere in both lungs are normal.

What has happened and how do all the patient's symptoms at this stage relate to her suspected diagnosis?

Answer 2

The majority of bronchial carcinomas develop as masses in the proximal bronchi, near to the hila of the lungs. As with other tubular structures and organs in the body, if a tumour develops, either from the mucosal lining of the tube or from the deeper tissues of the wall, the tube may become partially or completely obstructed by the neoplasm. Narrowing of a bronchus impedes air flow in and out of the part of the lung distal to that airway. If the volume of lung affected is sufficiently great, this can manifest as dyspnoea, especially in a patient who has COPD and therefore has decreased lung function anyway. In extreme cases, the obstruction is complete and causes collapse of the affected part of the lung. The findings in this patient on presentation suggested an element of collapse.

If a region of the lung is obstructed, the drainage of mucus and other airway secretions from that lung is impaired. Stagnant fluid is an advantageous environment for bacteria and they can colonize the fluid. In the lung, this leads to pneumonia in the occluded region. The immune system reacts with an acute inflammatory response, leading to the generation of pus which is coughed up as purulent sputum.

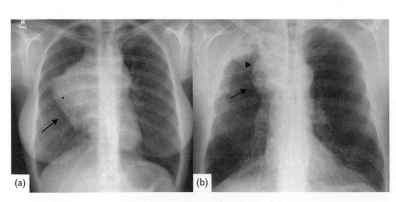

(a) (b)

Figure 6.1 (a) Chest X-ray showing right hilar and anterior mediastinal mass (arrow) – small cell lung cancer. (b) Chest X-ray showing right apical (arrowhead) and paramediastinal mass (arrow) invading the mediastinum – non-small cell lung cancer.

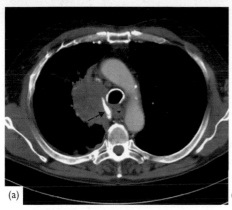
(a)

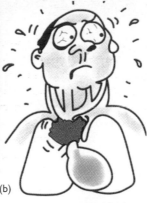
(b)

Figure 6.2 (a) CT scan showing lung cancer (red arrow) invading the mediastinum and compressing the superior vena cava (blue arrow) which is narrowed to a slit. (b) Obstruction of the superior vena cava is a medical emergency. Patients present with severe headache and congestion of veins in the face and upper body. The main differential diagnosis is from mediastinal tumours such as lymphoma. Thrombosis of cavernous sinus and veins draining the brain may cause death.

Extension of the pneumonic process to the pleura induces inflammation there. Movement of the inflamed parietal pleura over the visceral pleura produces pain.

Haemoptysis may result from two mechanisms. In addition to its ability to obstruct the lung, a bronchial carcinoma can also ulcerate the bronchial mucosa and will invade deeper structures. This damage may be accompanied by small quantities of blood loss. The other process that generates haemoptysis is cavitation. Malignant tumours are frequently rapidly growing and in some instances grow faster than their ability to induce adequate angiogenesis. When this happens, part of the tumour becomes necrotic and may undergo cavitation. This destructive collapse can be accompanied by haemorrhage.

It should be emphasized that a patient with COPD who presents with a cough that is productive of purulent sputum would normally be considered to have an infective exacerbation of their COPD. However, this would be accompanied by widespread wheeze in both lungs.

Question 3

In addition to obstructing the bronchus, or infiltrating the underlying lung, where else may a bronchial carcinoma invade and what clinical features can result?

Answer 3

Centrally placed tumours have access to the mediastinum and the assorted structures therein. These structures can be affected either by direct invasion or pressure effects.

- Damage to the left recurrent laryngeal nerve will lead to a unilateral vocal cord palsy, which will present as hoarseness or an altered voice.

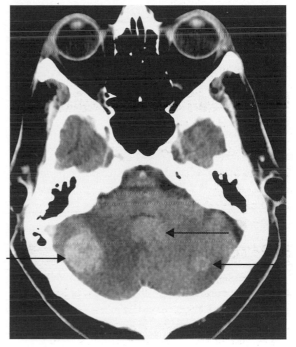

Figure 6.3 CT showing brain metastases (arrows) from a small cell lung cancer.

- Damage to the phrenic nerve will produce a unilateral diaphragmatic paralysis and a raised hemidiaphragm. Rarely, this may be the first presentation, via a chest X-ray, of a bronchial neoplasm.
- Invasion or compression of the superior vena cava obstructs the vessel, leading to vascular congestion of the head, neck and arms, coupled with the presence of dilated, superficial, collateral veins over the chest (Figure 6.2).
- Extension into the pericardium can produce a pericardial effusion. Pericardial and/or cardiac invasion

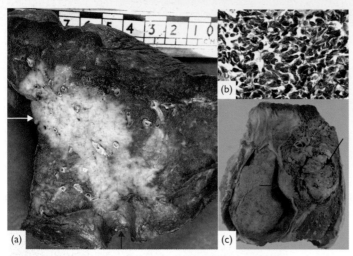

Figure 6.4 (a) Slice of lung infiltrated by tumour with invasion of the pleural (red arrow) and mediastinal (white arrow) surfaces. (b) Microscopic image of small cell lung carcinoma showing crushed blue cells with virtually no cytoplasm, previously called 'oat cell carcinoma' because of the cells' resemblance to heaps of oat grains and their propensity to scatter widely throughout the body. (c) Parasagittal view of a bronchial carcinoma (black arrow) invading anteriorly into the posterior aspect of the pericardium (red arrow). The heart is seen within the pericardial cavity.

may also cause atrial fibrillation, other arrhythmias or cardiac dysfunction.

- The oesophagus can be invaded or compressed, yielding dysphagia.

A tumour that is situated in the apex of the lung can extend upwards into the lower aspects of the brachial plexus. This is the Pancoast tumour and produces its initial neurological symptoms in the distribution of the C8 and T1 nerve roots, including their sympathetic component. This results in weakness of the small muscles of the hand, paraesthesia in the C8 and T1 dermatomes, and an ipsilateral Horner syndrome.

Peripherally situated carcinomas can invade into the pleura and cause a pleural effusion.

Question 4

Returning to the patient, she attends the local thoracic medicine clinic at which a chest X-ray reveals a right hilar mass. A CT scan and bronchoscopy are arranged. The CT scan is performed first and discloses enlarged mediastinal lymph nodes and an adrenal mass that is compatible with a metastasis. The brain is noted to be normal (unlike that shown in Figure 6.3).

When the patient attends for the bronchoscopy, she reports a new symptom of weakness in her lower limbs that is making it difficult to walk and particularly awkward to rise from a chair. To a lesser extent, she has also noticed that her arms are weaker.

The bronchoscopy confirms the presence of an obstructing, ulcerating tumour in the right lower lobe main bronchus. The biopsy shows the tumour to be a small cell carcinoma.

Given that the patient does not appear to have any cerebral or spinal metastases that would explain her neurological symptoms, how could they nevertheless be related to the tumour?

Answer 4

The patient has a paraneoplastic syndrome, in this case either Eaton–Lambert syndrome or (dermato)myositis.

A paraneoplastic syndrome is one that is caused by the production of a humoral agent by, or as a direct consequence of, the tumour, but is not due to the simple mass effect of the tumour. Small cell carcinomas are especially associated with paraneoplastic phenomena and this reflects their origin from neuroendocrine cells which can normally release active agents.

Eaton–Lambert syndrome is a rare disease in which there is an autoimmune response mounted against the presynaptic component of the neuromuscular junction that causes muscle weakness. Approximately 50 per cent of cases are paraneoplastic.

Dermatomyositis is also an autoimmune condition which has a strong association with the presence of an underlying neoplasm. The autoimmune response is directed against the skin and skeletal muscles, particularly those of the limb girdles. The cutaneous manifestations include the characteristic periorbital heliotrope rash.

This patient transpires to have Eaton–Lambert syndrome.

A 36-year-old man presents to accident and emergency with a 24-hour history of worsening cough, dyspnoea and fever. The cough is productive of yellow–green sputum that infrequently contains streaks of blood. He has previously been fit and well and is taking no medication. He has no allergies.

On examination, the patient's temperature is 38°C. His pulse is 110/minute and regular. The blood pressure is 115/75 mmHg. The jugular venous pressure (JVP) is not raised. The apex beat is undisplaced and normal. The heart sounds are normal and there are no added sounds or murmurs. Examination of the abdomen is unremarkable.

The patient's respiratory rate is 16/minute. He is able to talk in sentences and is not using his accessory muscles of respiration. No cyanosis is present. The trachea is central. Expansion is decreased on the right side and the patient reports a sharp pain in his chest when asked to breathe in deeply. The percussion note is dull at the right apex but resonant elsewhere. The breath sounds are bronchial at the right apex and vesicular elsewhere. There is also a harsh rubbing sound at the right apex. Oxygen saturations on room air are 99 per cent.

The patient's chest X-ray is shown in Figure 7.1.

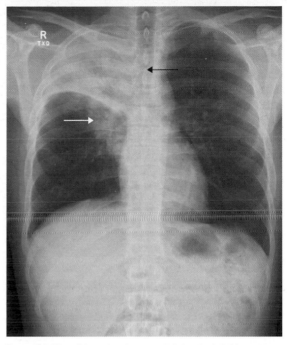

Figure 7.1 Chest X-ray showing consolidation in the right upper lobe (black arrow) and an enlarged right hilum due to reactive adenopathy (white arrow).

Question 1

What is the diagnosis and what pathological mechanism is involved?

Answer 1

The diagnosis is lobar pneumonia affecting the right upper lobe.

The pathological process is that of acute inflammation in response to bacterial infection, most commonly *Streptococcus pneumoniae*. While the major cell type involved in acute inflammation is the neutrophil, there is nevertheless a complex interplay of inflammatory cells and mediators. Most bacteria are potent inducers of an acute inflammatory response. Neutrophils and monocytes/macrophages are equipped to recognize and be stimulated by molecules in the bacterial cell wall. These molecules also trigger the complement system. Stimulation of these components of the acute inflammatory system initiates killing mechanisms and also recruits other cells into the fray, either by the release of assorted cytokines from the leukocytes, or by direct effects of activated complement.

Question 2

How does the acute inflammatory response explain the clinical and radiological changes in the lungs?

Answer 2

One of the characteristic features of a good-going acute inflammatory response is the development of pus, preceded in the initial stages by hyperaemia and oedema. In lobar pneumonia, this means that the air spaces of the affected lobe of the lung are filled with purulent fluid. The process by which the air spaces of the lung become filled with liquid is known as 'consolidation'.

The presence of fluid/pus in the lungs initiates a cough reflex. The cough is productive because the patient is expelling the pus, mixed with airway mucus, from the infected lobe.

The fluid in the alveoli and distal airways occupies the space that should have been filled with air. The

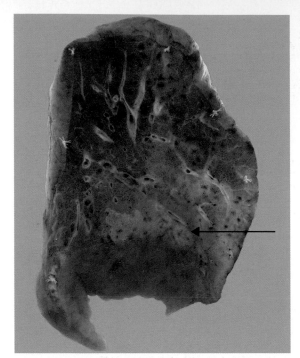

Figure 7.2 A vertical slice of lung showing consolidation in the lower lobe.

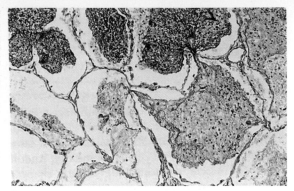

Figure 7.3 Photomicrograph of lung showing how lobar pneumonia develops as the fluid-rich inflammatory exudate spreads between alveolar spaces via spaces called 'pores of Kohn' (arrow).

Answer 3

Yes. Lobar pneumonia affects only one lobe of one lung and occurs in people who are otherwise fit and well and who have undamaged lungs. These people have sufficient lung function to absorb the loss of the gas transfer capacity of one lobe without impairing overall gaseous exchange.

Question 4

How is the condition likely to progress?

Answer 4

Lobar pneumonia is described as having four stages: acute congestion, red hepatization, grey hepatization and resolution. The first three reflect the establishment and peaking of the inflammatory response. The fourth, resolution, is one of the typical outcomes of acute inflammation.

The role of acute inflammation is to deal with a new insult, neutralize it and then to engage processes that clear up the mess. If this process operates with optimal results, the inflamed tissue or organ is restored back to normal, with no evidence that it was ever inflamed. Lobar pneumonia is one of the examples of an acute inflammatory condition that achieves this ideal result.

Acute inflammation in lobar pneumonia is initiated in order to destroy the invading bacteria. Once the neutrophils and complement systems have overcome the bacteria, the resulting dead cells and fluid need to be cleared from the airways. The simple and direct approach of coughing can remove the bulk of the consolidation, but macrophages are required to operate at the microscopic level to complete the clearing up

alveolar space, as with any hollow structure that it is filled with air, will produce a resonant note when percussed, but will be dull if occupied by a liquid or solid. The liquid also alters the quality of the breath sounds to give bronchial breathing. The reduced expansion of the affected lobe reflects the inability to inspire air into the involved air spaces to expand them because they are already filled with fluid and inflammatory debris.

The harsh rubbing sound is a pleural rub and is the counterpart of the sharp pain that the patient feels on inspiration. Both of these features indicate pleuritis, the process by which the inflammation extends to involve the pleura. Movement of the inflamed parietal pleura over the visceral pleura is painful, in part due to the various humoral inflammatory mediators released by the acute inflammatory system.

The chest X-ray findings echo the pathological changes. Liquid attenuates X-rays to a greater extent than air and thus the consolidated air spaces are relatively radio-opaque (Figure 7.2).

Question 3

The patient's gaseous exchange appears to be uncompromised. Is this plausible?

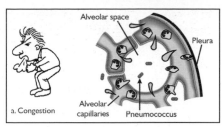

Acute congestion: bacteria invade alveolar spaces of lung. Acute inflammatory response characterized first by increased vascular permeability, with the formation of a fibrin-rich exudate

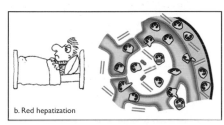

Red hepatization: neutrophils are quickly attracted to the site, accompanied by red blood cells. The fluid spreads between alveolar spaces via pores of Kohn and soon the entire lung lobe is consolidated (solidified) due to a mixture of fibrin, red and white blood cells. Neutrophils phagocytose the bacteria. The texture and colour of the lobe resemble fresh liver

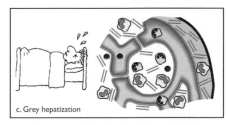

Grey hepatization: macrophages are attracted to the site, also lymphocytes. Further phagocytosis occurs. Bacteria and dead red and white cells are removed and the fibrin mesh starts to be digested. The grey/white colour of the lobe is due to the high fibrin and white cell content; the texture resembles cooked liver (ugh!)

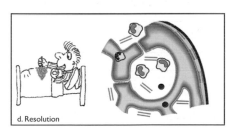

Resolution: the last few fibrin strands and white cells are removed, together with any remaining bacterial corpses and the lung returns to normal. This is possible because the basic skeleton of the lung (formed by reticulin, a type of collagen) is not damaged, unlike bronchopneumonia, in which the inflammatory process is centred on infected bronchioles and is characterized by destruction of the adjacent lung framework (this is usually followed by scarring of lung tissue)

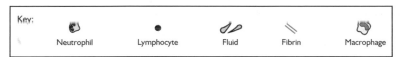

Key: Neutrophil   Lymphocyte   Fluid   Fibrin   Macrophage

Figure 7.4 The stages of lobar pneumonia.

process. Macrophages are versatile inflammatory cells and are particularly adept at removing debris.

In general, the affected lobe should have achieved normal reaeration by two to three weeks after the onset of the lobar pneumonia.

Question 5

Why does fever occur?

Answer 5

Numerous cytokines are released by inflammatory cells in acute inflammation and include assorted interleukins, prostaglandins and tumour necrosis factor. Among the numerous functions of these mediators is an action on the thermoregulatory centres of the hypothalamus to cause an elevation of body temperature. Although an unpleasant experience, fever is actually a beneficial response in infection because the increased body temperature impairs the replication of bacteria and viruses. The replication of microorganisms is dependent on enzyme function and modifications of temperature can interfere with enzymatic action. It has also been suggested that the increased body temperature of fever is helpful to various elements of the inflammatory system.

Question 6

Patients with lobar pneumonia and many other bacterial infections have an elevated white blood cell count that is due to an increase in the number of neutrophils. How and why does this occur?

Answer 6

Again, cytokines are responsible. Some of the inflammatory mediators released by an acute inflammatory response act on the progenitor cells of the bone marrow to stimulate the synthesis of mature neutrophils. Neutrophils are the frontline response to bacteria and even under peaceful circumstances they live for only five days. Once engaged in an inflammatory response, a neutrophil may survive for only a matter of minutes and most will be dead within 10 hours. Therefore, in order to maintain a supply of neutrophils to the inflammatory effort, the bone marrow must increase its output.

SUMMARY

Lobar pneumonia is an example of an acute inflammation. The trigger for the inflammation is a common one, bacterial infection.

Acute inflammation involves both cellular and humoral components. These act in a co-operative fashion. Many of the humoral components are secreted by the inflammatory cells and many of the humoral components modify the function of the inflammatory cells.

Most of the clinical features in lobar pneumonia are explained by the basic properties of acute inflammation. Blood flow increases to the affected lobe to bring neutrophils to the region and capillaries become more leaky to facilitate the entry of inflammatory cells and humoral mediators into the infected lobe. A cell-rich, protein-rich exudate rapidly accumulates and, once the killing of bacteria begins, purulent fluid soon gathers. This purulent fluid fills up the air spaces and is responsible for the cough and most of the clinical signs.

Nuala Fitzsimmons, aged 40 years, has been lacking in energy for the last few months. She has also had several episodes of abdominal pain. She consults her GP. On questioning she reveals that she has lost a few kilos in weight over the last few months.

Her past medical history is unremarkable, save for a hysterectomy aged 35 years following complications after the birth of her son, Conrad. He is a very small child, quite withdrawn and slightly miserable and takes a great deal of her attention.

The GP notes that she is pale and very slim, with no abnormality on systems examination. He requests a full blood count, which shows a normochromic, normocytic anaemia and normal platelet numbers. The GP refers her to a gastrointestinal physician at the local hospital.

Question 1

Explain the GP's reason for referring Nuala to a gastroenterologist rather than a haematologist.

Answer 1

Nuala is anaemic – the usual cause in premenopausal women is menorrhagia, not possible in her case. Abdominal pain and weight loss suggest a gastrointestinal problem.

Her GP wonders whether she might have coeliac disease giving her malabsorption, which is particularly prevalent in the Irish. The gastrointestinal physician recommends testing for coeliac antibodies and also that Nuala undergo an upper GI tract endoscopy.

Question 2

What is coeliac disease? What is the treatment?

Answer 2

Coeliac disease is caused by an immune reaction against the gliadin fraction of wheat protein, leading to inflammatory atrophy of the small bowel mucosa and malabsorption. The treatment is to change to a gluten-free diet.

Question 3

Why do some people have a genetic predisposition to develop coeliac disease? Who is at increased risk?

Answer 3

Those who inherit the MHC type II molecules HLA-DQ2 or -DQ8 have a predisposition to develop coeliac disease. These genotypes are common in the Irish but are prevalent throughout the world, with the exception of east Asia.

People with other autoimmune diseases (e.g. type 1 diabetes mellitus) are at increased risk of coeliac disease.

Curiously, coeliac disease may present at any age, from childhood to old age. Many people are thought to have subclinical disease (the 'coeliac iceberg'). It is possible that transiently increased gut permeability to larger protein molecules, possibly after infection, may precipitate coeliac disease in those who are genetically predisposed.

Nuala is negative on coeliac antibody testing.

Question 4

Which antibodies are useful in the diagnosis of coeliac disease?

Answer 4

Until relatively recently, serology for coeliac disease was limited to anti-gliadin antibodies. However, serology for anti-endomyseal (EMA) and anti-tissue transglutaminase (tTG) antibodies is now available. While anti-tTG is less specific than anti-EMA it is slightly more sensitive. Both have better sensitivity than anti-gliadin antibodies.

The detection of these antibodies is not diagnostic of coeliac disease. The incidence of anti-EMA in the Irish population is 1:100, but clinically manifest disease only exists in around 1:300. The corresponding figures for the rest of northern Europe are 1:300 and 1:1500.

As coeliac disease is a condition of a mucosal surface, the antibodies involved are often of the IgA type. However, about 4 per cent of patients with coeliac disease do not secrete IgA, compared with 0.4 per cent of the general population, so IgG antibodies, though less sensitive, are also sought.

Question 5

An upper gastrointestinal tract endoscopy is performed. The duodenum shows patchy red areas. The pathology report on the gastric and duodenal biopsies reads as follows:

> *The duodenal biopsies show patchy acute and chronic inflammation. Several loose, non-caseating granulomas are seen.*
>
> *The gastric biopsies show very occasional non-caseating granuloma formation.*
>
> *No parasites have been identified and a Ziehl–Neelsen stain for acid-fast bacilli is negative.*

What diagnoses are raised by these findings?

Answer 5

Granulomatous duodenitis and gastritis are not features of coeliac disease, which is characterized by diffuse villous atrophy, villous broadening by predominantly chronic inflammatory cells and a generalized increase in intraepithelial lymphocytes. The changes begin in the duodenum and extend along the jejunum, only rarely involving the terminal ileum.

In any patient with granulomas, the possibility of tuberculosis should be entertained. Despite the lack of

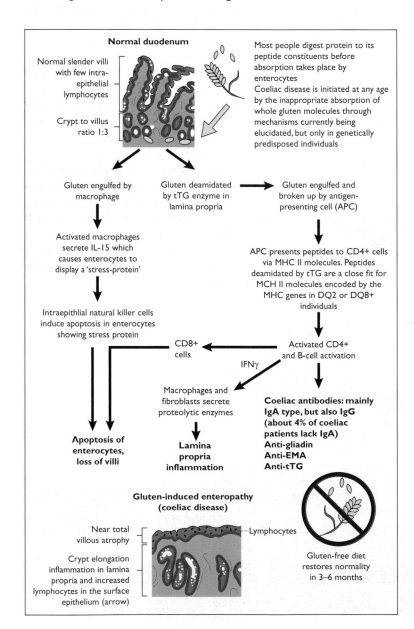

Figure 8.1 Coeliac disease: sensitivity to gliadin causes the typical histological features of coeliac disease: villous atrophy due to epithelial cell destruction, crypt hyperplasia due to expansion of epithelial cells in the proliferative compartment at the bases of the crypts, inflammation of the lamina propria and increased numbers of natural killer and CD8+ T cells in the epithelium.

caseation and the negative Ziehl–Neelsen stain, a Mantoux test and chest X-ray would be wise precautions. Note that caseation may not be seen and that acid-fast bacilli are often scanty and not visualized in tissue sections. Culture (for 6–12 weeks) may be necessary to maximize the chances of finding the organisms and establishing their drug sensitivities.

Taking the clinical picture as a whole, Crohn's disease should also be considered.

Nuala's Mantoux shows normal reactivity for a patient who has had BCG (bacille Calmette–Guérin) immunization and her chest X-ray is clear. She is advised that the tests have raised the possibility of Crohn's disease and undergoes a colonoscopy. This shows focal aphthous-type ulceration in the terminal ileum, but the colon is clear. At the anus, a small skin tag is noted and removed.

The pathology report reads as follows:

Focal superficial ulceration and acute inflammation are noted in the terminal ileum. In addition, several small non-caseating granulomas are noted in the mucosa and submucosa of the ileum and in the perianal skin tag, which is an inflamed fibroepithelial polyp. All the colonic and rectal biopsies appear normal.

Question 6

What is Crohn's disease and which part of the bowel does it usually affect?

Answer 6

Crohn's disease is an idiopathic chronic inflammatory bowel disease, which typically relapses and remits. It usually presents at puberty.

Crohn's disease typically affects the terminal ileum, and in two-thirds of patients there is patchy ileal involvement. However, any part of the gastrointestinal tract may be affected, and recurrent aphthous mouth ulceration, and oesophageal, gastric and duodenal inflammation are sometimes encountered.

Around 75 per cent of Crohn's patients have some form of perianal pathology — simple fibroepithelial polyps, granulomatous polyps or perianal fistulae and abscess formation being typical.

The disease may present with problems due to stricture formation, ulceration or fistula formation. If the colon is involved, the features may strongly resemble ulcerative colitis. If the ileum is the main site of involvement, malabsorption or obstructive problems may occur due to the formation of fibrotic strictures.

Over the next few days Nuala develops increasingly severe and persistent abdominal pain with signs of small intestinal obstruction: severe griping, colicky, abdominal pain, absent bowel sounds, and nausea and vomiting. She is admitted as an emergency.

A laparotomy is performed. The surgeon removes two thickened segments of small intestine: a rubber

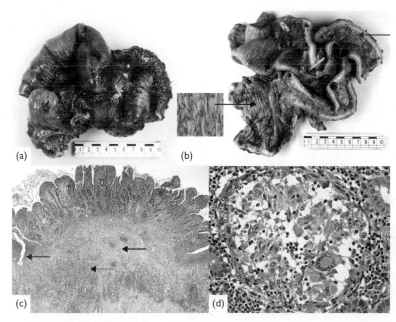

Figure 8.2 Crohn's disease. (a) Adherent loops of small bowel. (b) The specimen has been opened to show patchy, cobblestone-type ulceration (red arrow) and a focus of aphthous ulceration (blue arrow and inset). (c) Low-power microscope image shows fissuring ulcers (red arrow) and patchy transmural chronic inflammation (blue arrows). (d) Medium-power image shows a non-caseating granuloma.

hosepipe-like segment at the ileocaecal valve and two adherent loops of small bowel.

The pathology report reads:

The gross specimen shows adherent loops of small bowel exhibiting 'fat-wrapping' by mesenteric fat over the serosal surface. On opening, the ileal mucosa shows ulceration and oedema resembling cobblestone paving and the wall is 16 mm thick (normal 4 mm). Mesenteric lymph nodes are enlarged.

Microscopy shows patchy transmural chronic inflammation, with a 'beaded' pattern of lymphoid follicles outside muscularis propria, in serosal fat. Deep fissuring ulceration extends from the luminal surface into muscularis propria. The rest of the mucosa is normal. There are numerous non-caseating granulomas throughout the ileal wall and in occasional lymph nodes.

The loops of adherent small bowel are linked by a fistula track which is lined by granulation tissue.

Question 7

Summarize the typical gross and histological features of Crohn's disease described in this specimen.

Answer 7

Gross features: fat-wrapping (encroachment of mesenteric fat over the serosal surface) of the small bowel, patchy disease, fistula formation between loops of bowel, cobblestone mucosal appearance, patchy disease ('skip' lesions, with intervening normal mucosa).

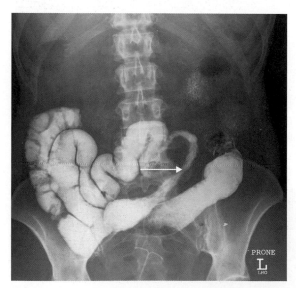

Figure 8.3 Small bowel follow-through study showing a mid-ileal stricture (arrow) in a patient with Crohn's disease.

Microscopic features: patchy chronic inflammation through the whole wall, granulomas, fissuring ulcers (resembling knife cuts) deep into the wall.

Question 8

Crohn's disease is an inflammatory bowel disease of unknown aetiology. It most often involves the small intestine, but about one-third of patients with Crohn's disease only have colonic disease. How does Crohn's disease differ from ulcerative colitis, the other important type of idiopathic inflammatory bowel disease?

Answer 8

- Crohn's disease usually involves the ileum but may occur in any part of the gastrointestinal tract and is patchy. If it affects the colon, it is usually proximal (right-sided).
- Ulcerative colitis involves only the colon, beginning in the rectum and extending proximally in a confluent fashion.
- Crohn's disease is characterized by mesenteric fat-wrapping, seen more in the ileum.
- Strictures and fistulae are typical of Crohn's disease, not seen in ulcerative colitis.
- Ulcerative colitis is a mucosal disease, affecting deeper layers only if there is ulceration of mucosa over a broad front, accompanied by fulminant colitis.
- Crohn's disease is transmural, with patchy lymphoid aggregates and deep, fissuring ulcers.
- Granulomas are typical of Crohn's disease, not ulcerative colitis. Currently there is no irrefutable proof of a single causative organism for either disease and it is more likely that they are caused by aberrant immune responsiveness to bacterial stimulation in the intestines.

Nuala recovers well after surgery. She is warned that the disease is one that relapses and remits and that during attacks she will need medication with steroids, other immunosuppressants and possibly anti-TNF drugs. Her surgeon warns her that she runs the risk of developing severe problems due to malabsorption, such as osteomalacia and other vitamin deficiencies if the disease continues to involve her duodenum and small bowel. She takes vitamin supplements in addition to her Crohn's medication. The surgeon warns her that her son may require investigation since inflammatory bowel disease can be familial. Her son's growth and development will be monitored closely.

A 34-year-old woman goes to see her GP because she is troubled by a collection of symptoms. She has noticed that over the past few months her face has become rounder and that her cheeks have become redder. In particular, she is perturbed by the development of a small quantity of facial hair. She has put on weight around her abdomen but is puzzled by this because her upper arms seem to be thinner despite the fact that she takes regular exercise (although she has found this harder to do since the problems began). The patient has also remarked on a tendency to bruise easily.

Further questioning reveals that the patient's menstrual cycle, which was previously stable and regular, has now become irregular. She also relates that some of her friends have told her that she has become more 'stroppy' recently. Overall, she does not feel in good health and is concerned that something serious is wrong.

Examination confirms the physical features that the patient has already described, as well as revealing a fat pad on the upper aspect of the back and neck. The patient's blood pressure is 165/92 mmHg.

Question 1

What is the probable diagnosis?

Answer 1

The patient is very likely to have Cushing's syndrome. The collection of clinical features is characteristic.

Question 2

What is the nature of this condition?

Answer 2

Cushing's syndrome is a condition in which there is persistent, inappropriate elevation of the levels of circulating corticosteroids.

Question 3

What metabolic disturbances could be present that the GP could ascertain with simple blood tests that day?

Answer 3

Corticosteroids have a variety of actions on metabolism. In Cushing's syndrome, these effects are exaggerated.

Many patients with Cushing's syndrome have secondary diabetes mellitus due to the prohyperglycaemic effects of steroids on glucose metabolism. The related actions on lipid metabolism account for the central fat deposition that is seen in Cushing's syndrome.

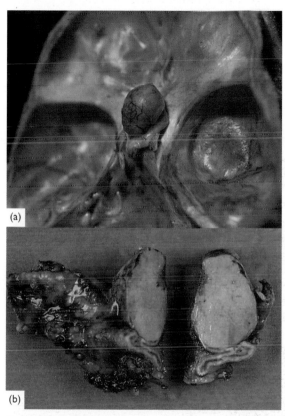

Figure 9.1 (a) Pituitary adenoma: view of base of skull. The enlarged pituitary protrudes from the surface – normally it is hidden inside the invaginated sella turcica. (b) Adrenocortical adenoma. It is bright yellow, reflecting the cholesterol core of the steroid hormones.

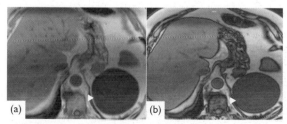

Figure 9.2 Axial in-phase (a) and out-of-phase (b) MRI. This technique relies on the fact that lipid-containing lesions drop in signal on the out-of-phase sequence. The MRI shows that the adrenal lesion contains fat and is therefore a lipid-rich adenoma. Note the renal cyst (arrowhead).

A minor derangement of electrolyte levels can be encountered in Cushing's syndrome. This is due to the natural, but weak, mineralocorticoid properties of glucocorticoids. In Cushing's syndrome, the elevated levels of glucocorticoids may be sufficient to permit them to exert a tangible aldosterone-like action. Hence, there can be hyperkalaemia and hyponatraemia, both usually of a mild degree.

In general, glucocorticoids function to elevate blood glucose and to mobilize fat and amino acids, especially from the periphery. This mobilization of proteins and lipids from the periphery (to an extent towards the central organs and tissues) can explain many of the clinical features, including easy bruising due to skin fragility and muscle weakness secondary to muscle protein loss.

Question 4

How could the secondary diabetes mellitus interact with another aspect of Cushing's syndrome?

Answer 4

Patients with Cushing's syndrome have a degree of immunosuppression due to the immunosuppressive actions of corticosteroids. There is also relatively mild immunocompromise in diabetes mellitus. These two processes may reinforce each other.

Question 5

What are the causes of Cushing's syndrome?

Answer 5

This question can be answered by considering the normal regulation of corticosteroid production. Corticosteroids are synthesized by the adrenal cortex in response to stimulation by ACTH (adrenocorticotrophic hormone) that is released by the anterior pituitary. Therefore, Cushing 's syndrome can result from any disease which:

- increases ACTH synthesis by the pituitary
- provides an aberrant source of ACTH outside the pituitary
- enables the adrenal glands to produce corticosteroids autonomously
- provides a source of corticosteroids outside the adrenal glands.

This basic principle also applies to other endocrine hyperfunction syndromes.

Thus, the answers are:

- ACTH-secreting pituitary tumour (Cushing's disease (see below))
- other ACTH-secreting tumour (e.g. small cell carcinoma of the lung)
- excess corticotrophin-releasing hormone (CRH) secretion (rare)
- adrenal adenoma
- adrenal carcinoma
- nodular adrenal hyperplasia
- exogenous steroids
- McCune–Albright syndrome.

Chronic alcohol excess can induce a pseudo-Cushing's appearance.

Question 6

What is the difference between Cushing's syndrome and Cushing's disease?

Answer 6

Cushing's disease is a particular cause of Cushing's syndrome in which the syndrome is due to a pituitary tumour that secretes ACTH.

Question 7

How could the diagnosis of Cushing's syndrome be confirmed?

Answer 7

The simple answer of doing a random cortisol level is not that helpful. Cortisol levels vary widely throughout

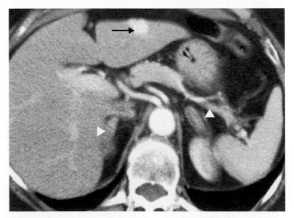

Figure 9.3 Axial CT post contrast showing bilateral adrenal hyperplasia (arrowheads). Note the haemangioma in the liver (arrow).

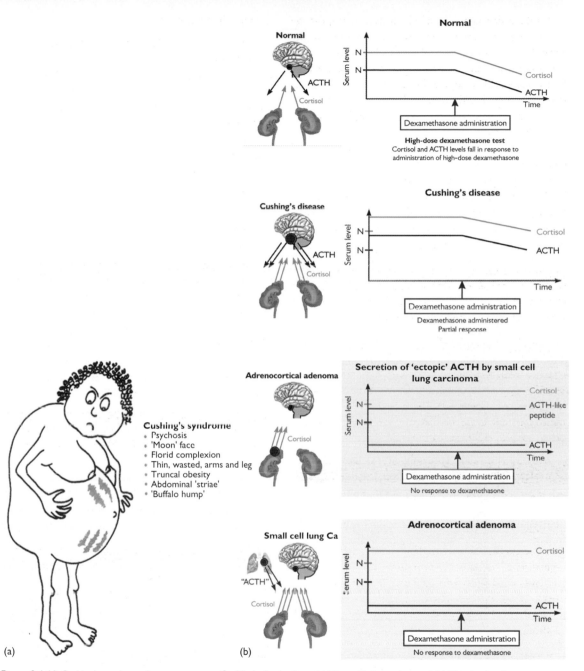

Figure 9.4 (a) Cushing's syndrome has many causes. Cushing's disease is caused by a pituitary adenoma. (b) The dexamethasone suppression test can help to identify the underlying problem. The principles of the test are shown here.

the day due to a natural circadian rhythm and as cortisol is a stress hormone they can also be affected by numerous other factors. All of this means that interpreting a single cortisol level is problematic because it is difficult to establish what the normal range should be. Nevertheless, there are situations in which a single cortisol level can be of use in guiding things in the right direction (for example, a very low level would be unusual except in exogenous corticosteroid administration).

The mainstay of the confirmation of the diagnosis is the dexamethasone suppression test (Figure 9.4b). This operates on the principle that, in the normal individual, the administration of a high dose of exogenous corticosteroids, in the form of dexamethasone, will suppress the endogenous secretion of corticosteroids by suppression of the pituitary–ACTH–adrenal axis. However, in Cushing's syndrome, this normal homeostatic pathway is non-functional and the administration of dexamethasone will have no effect on the autonomous and aberrant secretion of corticosteroids by the adrenal gland.

Question 8

What type of pituitary tumour produces ACTH?

Answer 8

An adenoma. This may either be a microadenoma (under 10 mm) or a macroadenoma derived from the normal glandular cells of the anterior pituitary gland.

Question 9

Given that different pathological processes can produce Cushing's syndrome, how can the precise cause be determined?

Answer 9

This process can be difficult and the details are outside the scope of this book. However, ACTH levels will be suppressed in cases of an adrenal tumour due to feedback of the corticosteroids onto a normal pituitary, but will be raised in pituitary adenomas or ectopic ACTH secretion. However, the behaviour of the hypothalamic–pituitary–adrenal axis can be complex in disease states, especially when ectopic sources of ACTH are involved, so details of tests designed to stimulate each of the elements of this axis cannot be included here.

Many of the causes are due to underlying mass lesions, so imaging can be of use in finding a mass lesion, but pituitary microadenomas are more difficult to discern.

Question 10

Why is small cell carcinoma of the lung especially likely to secrete ACTH?

Answer 10

Small cell carcinoma of the lung is derived from bronchial neuroendocrine cells. These cells naturally have secretory functions. Therefore, when malignant transformation occurs, the resulting cells are already set up with the basic metabolism to secrete various hormonal agents and it requires less perturbation of their DNA (relative to other cells) for them to then release inappropriate agents.

SUMMARY

Cushing's syndrome is an example of an endocrine hyperactivity syndrome. Many of the clinical features can be predicted from knowledge of the normal physiological functions of the involved hormones.

The causes primarily centre around neoplasia and illustrate that a neoplasm, either benign or malignant, can retain some of the secretory functions of the tissue of origin. Furthermore, a neoplasm may acquire secretory functions that are not those of the underlying organ and yield a paraneoplastic syndrome.

After Saturday night had blurred into Sunday morning, which in turn had smeared, with the aid of abundant lubrication from alcohol, into Sunday evening and the lupine hours of the night, attendance at a Monday morning thoracic medicine outpatient clinic, complete with an eight o'clock start time, was one of the last things that Sarah McKenzie, a third-year medical student, needed. Unfortunately, her fatigued, hung-over and shattered state would count as no excuse with the professor of respiratory medicine, Roland Paul, and the prospect of having to repeat the six-week attachment was even more onerous to Sarah than the idea of having to leave the comfort of her bed that day. She did not even dare to entreat a little sympathy from the professor as he would be likely to regale her, plus any patient who was unfortunate enough to be captive in the consultation room, with a 45-minute anecdote regarding his antics as a medical student and how he had once

passed his fourth-year exams with flying colours despite having imbibed enough whiskey to render an elephant unconscious. Sarah wondered if these were the same fourth-year exams he had passed with similar distinction after having been knocked unconscious the previous day in scoring the winning try for his medical school's rugby team in the yearly showdown with their bitter rivals, or the same exams that had been negotiated with devastating aplomb despite having only recovered from meningitis five hours earlier.

Feeling like her inner ears were now so sensitive she could detect anybody stamping their foot within five miles, Sarah tentatively sat down in a chair outside the clinic to await the arrival of the professor. She tried to prepare herself to endure the tedious stream of tales of exploits, japes and triumphs with which the professor deemed it compulsory to torture his students, or to be able to maintain her concentration during one of his

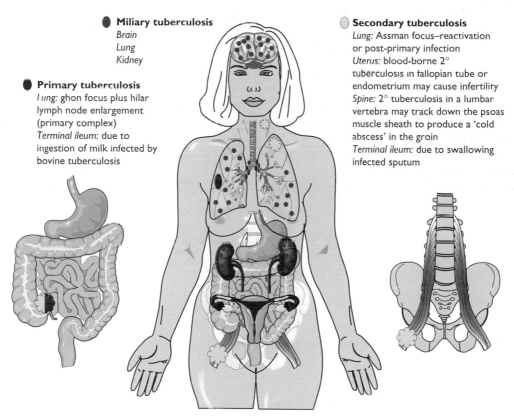

Miliary tuberculosis
Brain
Lung
Kidney

Primary tuberculosis
Lung: ghon focus plus hilar lymph node enlargement (primary complex)
Terminal ileum: due to ingestion of milk infected by bovine tuberculosis

Secondary tuberculosis
Lung: Assman focus—reactivation or post-primary infection
Uterus: blood-borne 2° tuberculosis in fallopian tube or endometrium may cause infertility
Spine: 2° tuberculosis in a lumbar vertebra may track down the psoas muscle sheath to produce a 'cold abscess' in the groin
Terminal ileum: due to swallowing infected sputum

Figure 10.1 Typical patterns of tuberculosis involvement in primary, secondary and miliary TB. Post-primary TB may be due to reactivation of old infection or new infection. Miliary TB may occur at any stage, if sufficient organisms are released into the blood.

interminable rambles for long enough to glean the one useful nugget of knowledge that was therein buried.

Professor Paul arrived punctually and beckoned Sarah into the consulting room with him. The first patient was a 29-year-old woman who had recently been diagnosed as having tuberculous lymphadenitis of a right neck lymph node and was attending to receive the diagnosis and to have her treatment explained to her.

Once the patient had left, Professor Paul embarked on a discourse about the history of tuberculosis, or, at least, that seemed to have been his intention when he began his oratory, but it meandered through his under-graduate career, his time as a research registrar and somehow managed to incorporate the moon landings, until finally, without any appropriate preceding con-text, he looked straight at Sarah and remarked 'Of course, if anybody asks you the clinical features of tuberculosis, you're laughing, because TB can cause anything. Historically, it has been known as the great mimic. You name it, TB can cause it. That said, if you don't start off with the pulmonary symptoms, I'd fail you in an exam, but that's by the by. Yes, the great mimic, can cause anything.'

Question 1

What is the underlying pathology of tuberculosis (TB) and how does this relate to the professor's assertion?

Answer 1a

Tuberculosis is an infection with the organism *Mycobacterium tuberculosis*. Other species of mycobact-eria also exist and are generally referred to as atypical mycobacteria or atypical TB.

Mycobacteria have the useful ability to be able to sur-vive phagocytosis. In normal phagocytosis, an organism is ingested by the phagocytic cell (e.g. a neutrophil or macrophage) which wraps its outer membrane around the organism to create a phagosome. Lysosomes con-taining toxic contents then fuse with the phagosome,

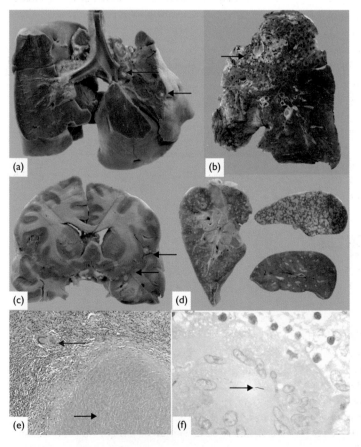

Figure 10.2 (a) The Ghon complex, primary tuberculosis of the lung, with a tiny peripheral focus (black arrow) and enlarged hilar lymph nodes (red arrow). Both areas show the white change typical of caseation necrosis. (b) Secondary or reactivation tuberculosis: a large cavity gapes open at the apex of the lung (arrow) and there are numerous foci of caseation necrosis in the adjacent lung tissue. (c) Tiny tuberculous nodules (arrows) are present along the meninges and focally within the adjacent brain tissue. (d) Miliary TB: tiny white nodules are scattered like millet seeds throughout the body – here we see a slice from a child's lung, liver and spleen. (e) Medium-power microscope image showing granular, amorphous caseation necrosis (black arrow), and a Langhans' giant cell (red arrow) with nuclei arranged in a horseshoe pattern at the periphery, H&E stain. (f) High-power view of acid-fast bacilli stained red by the Ziehl–Neelsen stain.

and the toxic contents kill the organism. Mycobacteria, however, can live in the phagosome and prevent the fusion of lysosomes with the phagosome and so they are protected from the toxic contents of the lysosome. This capacity of mycobacteria to survive phagocytosis renders neutrophils ineffective against them and requires macrophages to resort to other strategies.

Answer 1b

When faced with an organism or inanimate substance that resists normal phagocytosis, macrophages can become further activated to form giant cells. This process requires co-ordination by T lymphocytes and results in multiple macrophages fusing together to form a single giant cell that has multiple nuclei and the ability to handle more stubborn phagocytic targets.

In TB, the normal immune system reacts with a macrophage, giant cell and lymphocytic response. The macrophages form aggregates. The term 'granuloma' is employed for a collection of activated macrophages. Assorted diseases can cause granulomas to develop. The granulomatous response is accompanied by fibrosis. In the case of TB, the granulomas also exhibit the phenomenon of caseation. This is a type of necrosis that resembles cheese macroscopically. Although it is highly characteristic of TB, it is not pathognomonic for it. The presence of granulomas and fibrosis within an organ results in the replacement of normal tissue, particularly if there is the accompanying destructive element of caseous necrosis. In addition, the cytokine production that is part of the granulomatous response may also have effects on adjacent tissue. This damage to an organ causes a disruption of its function and, given that TB can infect virtually any organ in the body, it follows that TB can produce features in any of these organs.

Question 2

Which organ is most typically affected by TB and how are the usual symptoms of cough and haemoptysis explained?

Answer 2

The lung is the typical site of infection by TB. The initial, primary infection is often asymptomatic and consists of a small focus in the periphery of the lung and accompanying hilar lymphadenopathy. In a person with a healthy immune system, the body is able to contain the initial infection with the granulomatous and fibrotic response, in effect incarcerating the mycobacteria and preventing them from spreading. This can occur with sufficiently little organ damage so that it is asymptomatic, or presents only as a cold-like illness.

Secondary TB develops when the primary infection reactivates, or if a second infection occurs. The precise factors that determine why reactivation happens are uncertain in many people, although a degree of immune suppression, such as the use of corticosteroids, is relevant in some. Secondary TB preferentially affects the apices of the lung, possibly due to better aeration in this zone. The granulomatous and fibrotic process once again occurs, but this time does not so readily contain the organisms. Instead, there is fibrosis of the affected apices, sometimes with destruction of lung tissue and cavitation and thereby haemoptysis. The ongoing inflammation within the interstitium triggers coughing, but as TB is not usually accompanied by the generation of pus, which is a neutrophil response, the cough is typically fairly dry.

Depending on the particular virulence of the strain of TB and the constitution of the host, the secondary infection may ultimately be controlled, or may gradually progress, leading to more widespread pulmonary damage and disease in other organs.

Question 3

What problems could occur in somebody who has defective cell-mediated immunity?

Answer 3

Functioning cell-mediated immunity is vital to generate an effective granulomatous response. If this is absent, the immune system cannot fight the mycobacteria effectively. In severe cases, this results in miliary TB, in which a myriad of small foci of infection, likened to millet seeds, are scattered throughout various organs, especially the lungs, liver and spleen. In less marked cases of immunosuppression, the patient suffers from an increased susceptibility to TB, without necessarily developing miliary TB.

Patients with defective cell-mediated immunity are also susceptible to infection with atypical mycobacteria that would not normally be pathogenic.

Question 4

Once she had escaped from the outpatient clinic and her head had been liberated from the consequences of the weekend, Sarah wondered if there were any other diseases that had the property of being able to cause most clinical features in most organ systems. What are these diseases and what are their mechanisms of action?

Answer 4

Tuberculosis illustrates the granulomatous and fibrotic process as a cause of anything. There are two other main mechanisms by which a disease can produce almost any given clinical feature. The first is the vasculitic process. A vasculitis can cause organ ischaemia and organ dysfunction and, as most organs in the body depend upon a blood supply to operate, they are vulnerable to vasculitis. The second process is neoplasia. The simple mass effects of a tumour and its metastases can cause many clinical features and paraneoplastic phenomena can often fill in any gaps that are left. This yields the following list:

- systemic vasculitis
- systemic lupus erythematosus (SLE)
- syphilis
- sarcoidosis
- tuberculosis
- neoplasia – mass effect and paraneoplastic.

Systemic lupus erythematosus is primarily a vasculitic (and immune complex) – mediated disease. Syphilis and sarcoidosis are granulomatous, but can also demonstrate a vasculitic component.

The list must also be supplemented with amyloidosis (abnormal protein deposition) and drugs. (Idiopathic can be appended, although might be considered to be a form of tautology and stating congenital as a cause requires an ability to discuss the specific syndromes.)

Other than bailing people out in exams, the practical value of this list is in guiding management when dealing with a patient whose presentation does not fit any typical diagnosis. Consideration of the above conditions will address many serious diseases that could be amenable to treatment if recognized, but for which failure to identify them could have significant consequences.

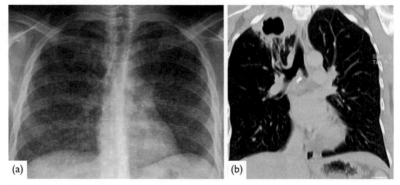

(a)   (b)

Figure 10.3 (a) Chest X-ray showing fine nodules throughout both lungs (nodules you would have to pick with a tweezer) in a patient with miliary TB. (b) Coronal CT showing a cavitating lesion at the right lung apex – secondary reactivation of TB.

PART 2

SIGNS

A 32-year-old woman attends the neurology outpatient department for her first follow-up appointment. Her history is somewhat detailed and features several separate episodes.

The initial presentation was five months previously with pins and needles in her left foot. This subsided after a few days and at the time the patient attributed it to having slept in an awkward position. However, six weeks later she noticed clumsiness in her right hand which was not of a severe degree, but was sufficient to interfere with her ability to play the piano and prompted her to consult her GP. By the time of the appointment, the clumsiness had resolved. However, the doctor did find a right upgoing plantar reflex on examination.

Her GP arranged referral to the local neurology outpatient clinic. In the three weeks while waiting for the date of the appointment, the patient suffered visual loss in her right eye. She noticed this on waking up in the morning but had been aware of a dull ache in her eye just before she went to bed. The patient went straight to accident and emergency where assessment revealed marked loss of visual acuity in her right eye such that she could perceive only light and dark. No vascular lesions were found in the retina on fundoscopy, although the optic disc was swollen. Intraocular pressure was normal and the left eye was normal, including the visual fields.

The patient was seen by the neurologists at this juncture. Neurological examination disclosed a mild increase in tone in the left upper limb, although power was normal.

The neurologists organized several investigations including a lumbar puncture, visual evoked potentials and MRI of the brain and spinal cord. The patient's vision returned to normal in the right eye after a week.

In the interval between the initial consultation and the first follow-up appointment, the patient suffered a further episode of pins and needles in her left foot. On this occasion she found that the pins and needles became worse if she flexed her neck.

On the day of her follow-up appointment, the patient noticed weakness of her right arm. This became worse when she left the house and improved a little when she entered the hospital. The only factor to which she could attribute this transient exacerbation was that it was a very hot day outside, while her house was well ventilated and cool and the hospital had effective air conditioning. On examination, she had grade 4/5 power throughout her right upper limb in conjunction with hypertonia and hyperreflexia. There was no wasting and no abnormal movements. Sensation and co-ordination were intact.

Question 1

Can the patient's symptoms and signs be explained by a single focal lesion?

Answer 1

No. Even if the sensory features are put to one side in order to avoid a lengthy discussion of the anatomy of the various sensory pathways, the patient has clinical features that have affected the following structures:

- Somatosensory for left half of the body: paraesthesia in left foot
- Right cerebellar hemisphere: clumsiness in the right hand
- Left corticospinal tract arising from the left cerebral hemisphere: right upgoing plantar; possible contribution to clumsiness (weakness may impair function)
- Right optic nerve: loss of vision in the right eye
- Right corticospinal tract: increased tone in left arm
- Left corticospinal tract again: weakness of right arm.

No plausible single mass or vascular lesion could involve all of these anatomical sites.

Question 2

What is the term used to describe the motor problem in the patient's right arm that was present when she attended the outpatient department for her follow-up appointment?

Answer 2

The patient has an upper motor neurone lesion.

The motor system is organized into upper and lower motor neurones. Lesions of the upper or lower motor neurone system produce characteristic clinical features (Table 11.1), most of which can be predicted from the normal physiology and pathophysiology.

Table 11.1 Features of upper and lower motor neurone lesions

	Upper motor neurone	Lower motor neurone
Inspection	No wasting (until late)	Wasting and fasciculations
Posture	Spastic – flexor movements dominate in upper limb and extensor in the lower	No specific features, contractures in late disease
Tone	Increased	Decreased
Power	Decreased	Decreased
Reflexes	Increased	Decreased or absent
Plantars	Upgoing	Downgoing

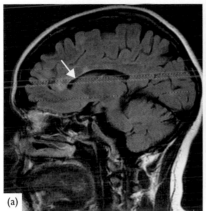

(a)

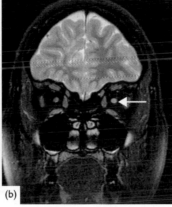

(b)

Figure 11.1 (a) Sagittal FLAIR MRI sequence showing the presence of demyelinating plaques (arrow) in the deep white matter of the right hemisphere. (b) Optic neuritis in multiple sclerosis with an asymmetrically bright left optic nerve (arrow) – coronal T2-weighted sequence through the orbit.

The lower motor neurone is the ultimate and sole output pathway for the brain and spinal cord to send a signal to the skeletal muscle. If the lower motor neurone is severed, communication between the nervous system and the muscle is lost and so is voluntary movement. In addition, the reflex arc is broken, so reflexes are reduced or lost. Loss of the lower motor neurone (and reflex arc) deprives the muscle of the basal stimulus that maintains tone, so tone is decreased. Loss of this basal stimulus to the muscle also results in atrophy due to disuse. Fasciculations are more complex to explain, but in simple terms may be considered to be caused by ineffective attempts by the surviving lower motor neurones to innervate muscle fibres that have lost their original nerve supply.

The upper motor neurones are situated in the primary motor cortex and their axons form the cortiospinal tract. This is the output station for voluntary movement commands generated by the brain. If the upper motor neurone is disrupted, the brain loses this output pathway and voluntary movement is lost. However, the local reflex arc remains intact and thus wasting tends not to occur until very late after the onset of the upper motor neurone lesion because the muscle receives some basal stimulation via the reflex arc and spinal reflex systems. The increase in tone, hyperreflexia and upgoing plantars that are encountered in upper motor neurone lesions reflect the fact that much of the basal activity in the descending upper motor neurone (corticospinal) pathway is actually inhibitory. This inhibitory input onto the lower motor neurone system is intended to suppress primitive spinal reflex arcs and motor systems that have a useful function in simpler animals but need to be overridden in humans to permit complex voluntary movement. (Very young babies demonstrate an ineffective stepping reflex if held upright. This is soon lost because far more complex patterns of movement are required for upright bipedal gait.)

Question 3

Do the patient's clinical features seem to reflect one single event in time, or events at separate points in time?

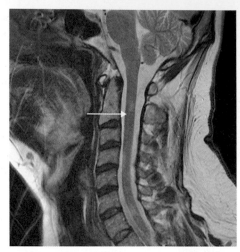

Figure 11.2 Demyelinating plaque in the spinal cord (arrow). MRI used in conjunction with cerebrospinal fluid analysis, electrophysiological studies and clinical presentation aids in the diagnosis of multiple sclerosis. MRI is also used to document the progress of the disease and to assess the effect of therapeutic interventions.

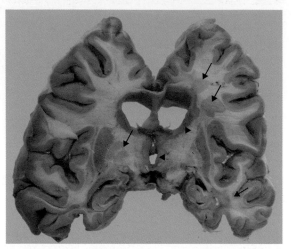

Figure 11.4 Coronal slice of the cerebral hemispheres in which several chronic plaques (arrows), which appear as sharply defined grey lesions of demyelination, are observed within the white matter. Acute lesions appear pink and ill defined (arrowheads).

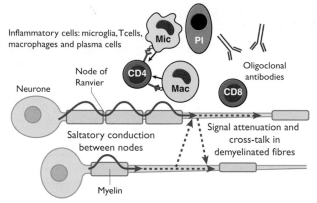

Figure 11.3 Multiple sclerosis is a form of autoimmune disease in which T cells attack myelin – the initial stimulus for this is as yet not clear. T cells are not usually present in the brain, because of the blood–brain barrier. A putative explanation is that an initial inflammatory stimulus in the brain (e.g. viral infection) attracts lymphocytes and macrophages to the site following upregulation of endothelial adhesion molecules in cerebral blood vessels by cytokines released by the brain's macrophages, the microglial cells. CD4 cells co-ordinate the response. CD8 cells predominate in the plaques and plasma cells secrete a small range of antibodies to myelin epitopes which can be detected in the cerebrospinal fluid.

Answer 3

The history indicates events that are separated in time. Hence, the patient has a process in which there are lesions that are disseminated in time as well as space.

Question 4

The MRI scan revealed several lesions in the periventricular white matter, as well as one in the white matter of the right cerebellar hemisphere. The visual evoked potentials for the right eye demonstrated a conduction delay. Oligoclonal bands were found in the patient's cerebrospinal fluid but no infection. Blood tests revealed no evidence of a vasculitic or infective process. What is the diagnosis?

Answer 4

The patient has multiple sclerosis.

Question 5

How is the disease defined?

Answer 5

Multiple sclerosis is a condition of likely autoimmune aetiology in which there are lesions of demyelination within the central nervous system (CNS) that are disseminated in time and space (in the absence of another cause). (Conditions that may mimic multiple sclerosis include vasculitis, systemic lupus erythematosus and Lyme disease.)

Question 6

What is the normal function of myelin?

Answer 6

Myelin insulates axons. This insulation greatly limits loss of the electrical signal as it is conducted along the axon, increases conduction velocity and prevents short-circuiting between adjacent fibres.

Question 7

What are the consequences of demyelination?

Answer 7

- The electrical impulse becomes dissipated as it attempts to pass along a demyelinated axon. This dissipation results in a weaker signal reaching the axon terminal or may be sufficient to block conduction altogether.
- Neuronal electrical conduction is slowed.
- Adjacent demyelinated axons can short-circuit, triggering unintentional activity.

- Demyelinated axons are susceptible to depolarization by mechanical trauma (such as stretching or flexing of the neck).
- An increase in temperature increases resistance in an axon and this can exacerbate the effects of demyelination.

Overall, the effect of demyelination is to disrupt the function of the demyelinated neuronal pathway. This can yield common effects such as straightforward upper motor neurone lesions or paraesthesia, or can produce more complex motor abnormalities if tracts relating to the basal ganglia system are involved. Not all lesions of demyelination in multiple sclerosis are clinically apparent.

Question 8

Why do the lesions sometimes improve in multiple sclerosis, giving the classical relapsing and remitting pattern?

Answer 8

This is not entirely clear, given that remyelination is often not fully accomplished. It has been suggested that some of the effects are mediated by the components of the autoimmune inflammatory response, such as oedema, and once these subside after the initial phase there is the potential for some recovery of function. Spare capacity within neuronal pathways may also allow a given system to absorb some damage but still function at normal levels, albeit with less reserve in the case of further injury.

A 76-year-old woman is brought to accident and emergency having had a sudden onset of weakness of her right arm and leg that is associated with difficulty in speaking and occurred 90 minutes earlier. The weakness was without warning or precipitating event. The patient's previous medical history is unremarkable other than a hysterectomy 30 years ago.

On examination, the cardiovascular, respiratory and abdominal systems are unremarkable. Examination of the limbs reveals normal power in the left arm and lower limb, but grade 0 power in the right arm and lower limb. There is hyperreflexia of the biceps, brachioradialis, triceps, knee and ankle reflexes on the right and the right plantar response is upgoing. Tone is increased on the right. There are no abnormal movements, fasciculations or wasting. Co-ordination is not assessable in the right limbs due to the loss of power, but is normal in the left arm and lower limb. Widespread sensory loss for all modalities is present in the right arm and lower limb.

Examination of the cranial nerves reveals a right homonymous hemianopia and weakness of the upper part of the right side of the face.

The patient understands verbal instructions, but has great difficulty in speaking and uses only short, incomplete sentences. She seems to be frustrated by her inability to speak. She is able to sip a glass of water without problems.

Question 1

What is the diagnosis?

Answer 1

The patient has had a cerebrovascular accident (CVA).

Question 2

What is the definition of a CVA?

Answer 2

A CVA is a focal, irreversible neurological deficit that persists for more than 24 hours and is due to a disruption to the blood supply of part of the brain.

Question 3

How does a CVA differ from a transient ischaemic attack (TIA)?

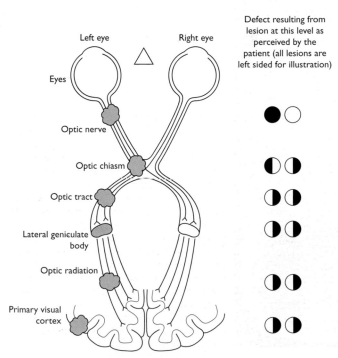

Figure 12.1 The effects on the visual fields of lesions at different levels in the visual pathway (visual field loss shown in black).

Answer 3

A TIA is fully reversible and the focal neurological deficit that is present lasts for no more than 24 hours. Typically a TIA resolves in a matter of minutes.

The 24-hour time-scale is the one employed to distinguish a TIA from a CVA in definition, but in clinical practice most patients whose symptoms have lasted for more than a few minutes, usually long enough for them to have reached hospital, will transpire to have had a CVA and so are diagnosed as such, even if the 24-hour time has not been reached. If treatment such as thrombolysis is intended, every minute saved is essential and waiting a day to meet the letter of the law would deprive the patient of any therapeutic benefit.

In the case of the reasoning behind the diagnosis in this patient, disruption of blood flow to the brain typically presents with a sudden onset of clinical features and her pattern of features is focal within a specific vascular territory of the brain.

Question 4

What are the two main types of CVA, what are the risk factors and which type has this patient had?

Answer 4

A CVA can be thromboembolic (around 80 per cent) or haemorrhagic (approximately 20 per cent).

In a thromboembolic CVA, the vessel is blocked by blood clot, whereas in a haemorrhagic one there is a bleed into the cerebral tissues. Most thromboembolic CVAs are associated with atherosclerosis and therefore have the same risk factors as other atherosclerotic conditions (such as angina or myocardial infarction). In addition, hypercoaguable states are also a risk factor. Embolic sources in the heart such as atrial or ventricular thrombus, vegetations and atrial myxomas should also be considered.

In haemorrhagic CVAs the main risk factor is hypertension. Coagulopathies may also be implicated.

This patient is likely to have had a thromboembolic CVA and this is confirmed on scanning. Haemorrhagic strokes are even more disruptive, patients often lose consciousness and they have a higher mortality.

Question 5

Why do CVAs yield focal deficits that affect specific neurological functions and why are they considered to be irreversible?

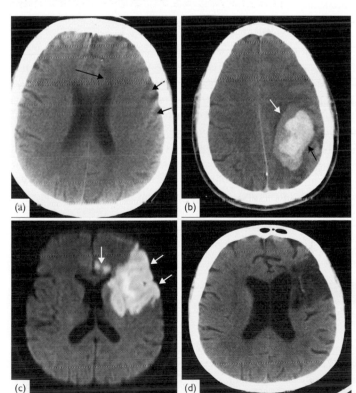

Figure 12.2 (a) Urgent CT on a man with an acute right hemiplegia. The CT shows subtle low density in the left middle cerebral territory (arrows) which could easily be missed. (b) CT scan in a different patient with acute right hemiplegia showing a haemorrhagic infarct in the left middle cerebral artery territory. Acute haemorrhage is bright on CT (arrow). (c) Another patient underwent urgent MRI within hours of a stroke. The image shows multifocal infarcts (arrows). This is diffusion-weighted imaging (DWI) – the bright areas reflect areas of restricted water movement – in effect mapping areas of cytotoxic oedema (dying or dead cells filled with water with nowhere to go). DWI scans can show infarcts within 2 hours of onset. (d) A CT scan on this patient 1–2 weeks later shows the area of infarction as a dark area with loss of volume in that part of the brain.

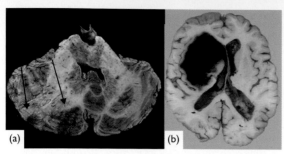

Figure 12.3 Gross appearances of (a) cerebellum with ischaemic stroke (arrows) and (b) axial brain with haemorrhagic stroke. The area involved is less well demarcated in (a), which shows multiple lesions, due to a shower of thromboemboli causing multiple infarcts.

Answer 5

Certain neurological functions such as motor control, sensation, speech, vision and co-ordination are consistently localized to specific parts of the brain in all individuals. The blood supply to different parts of the brain is also consistent between individuals. Therefore, disruption to the blood flow to a certain part of the brain will disrupt the function of that part of the brain, in many cases yielding a predictable neurological deficit.

Neurones have a very high metabolic demand and tolerate ischaemia very poorly. Within only a few minutes of the onset of ischaemia, neuronal cell death occurs and is irreversible. The capacity for cell division is extremely limited in mature neurones (until recently it was considered to be completely non-existent). Therefore, the dead neuronal tissue cannot be replaced with new neurones and any specialized function it served is lost. In addition, the adult brain tends to be much less adaptable than that of young children with regard to relearning fundamental motor and sensory pathways. Thus, while there can be some recovery of function after a CVA, by adaptation of unaffected parts of the brain, it is often limited, especially if the initial CVA yielded a pronounced deficit.

Question 6

Where in this patient's brain has the CVA occurred and in the territory of which blood vessel?

Answer 6

The CVA is in the left cerebral hemisphere. The combination of neurological defects indicates brain regions that are all located in the territory of the left middle cerebral artery.

Motor and sensory function displays right–left inversion in the cerebral hemispheres. Thus, the left cerebral hemisphere deals with motor and sensory function for the right side of the body and vice versa. By contrast, cerebellar hemisphere function is ipsilateral.

The overall visual field is split into a right and left half. Information from the right and left retina is divided at the optic chiasm into a left and right visual field by organizing the fibres from the temporal and nasal halves of each retina accordingly. As with motor and sensory function, the visual fields also exhibit left–right inversion. Thus, the left cerebral hemisphere deals with the right visual field and vice versa.

The lateralization of speech is slightly more complex. Over 99 per cent of right-handed people have their speech centres in the left cerebral hemisphere. The left cerebral hemisphere also contains the speech centres of more than 50 per cent of left-handed people.

Question 7

What is the term given to disruption to the patient's speech?

Answer 7

The patient has an expressive dysphasia.

Dysphasia is a higher disorder of language function in the cerebral hemisphere(s) while the basic physical structures required to produce speech (larynx, pharynx, tongue and other oral structures), plus the associated muscles and their innervation are intact. By contrast, in dysarthria the higher language function is intact and instead the neurological defect lies in the neuronal pathways that directly innervate these physical structures (such as the vagus nerve and its brainstem nucleus).

There are two main types of dysphasia and these reflect the organization of speech and language function within the brain.

- Broca's area is situated close to the inferior part of the primary motor cortex on the lateral aspect of the relevant cerebral hemisphere (usually the left). It deals with the motor aspect of generating fluent speech. A patient with a lesion that affects just Broca's area will understand language input but has difficulty producing fluent output. Their speech tends to focus on the key words and concepts of a sentence and conveys contextually appropriate meaning, but is not fluent or flowing.

- Wernicke's area is located in the temporal cortex close to the primary auditory cortex. It is concerned with understanding language and in organizing the grammar and content of language. A patient with a lesion that affects Wernicke's area will have difficulty in understanding any language input that is given to them and may therefore not be able to follow commands. Furthermore, although the speech they produce is flowing and may often be copious, grammar and syntax are lost and what the patient says is typically nonsense even though each word is normally formed.

If both areas are affected, the patient has a mixed dysphasia in which their comprehension of language is lost and their ability to speak is markedly impaired.

In addition, there is also a white matter tract that links Wernicke's area to Broca's area and relays the language output generated in Wernicke's area to Broca's region for conversion into motor patterns. Isolated lesions of this are unusual.

Interesting situations can arise in patients who have learnt a second language before the age of approximately five years. People who become bilingual at this early age generate a set of speech centres for each language. A small CVA may therefore disrupt one language but not the other. People who learn a second language at a later age usually employ their existing single set of speech centres.

Question 8

What macroscopic changes would be expected to be seen in an old cerebral infarct?

Answer 8

The process of necrosis in the brain is of the liquefactive type. Unlike other organs, the brain does not demonstrate a significant fibroblastic/fibrotic response to injury/infarction. Instead, the dead brain tissue, which has a very high water and fat content, is ingested by microglial cells and removed from the infarcted region. This removal without replacement by fibrous repair tissue results in a cystic cavity which fills with cerebrospinal fluid. The damaged grey and white matter is lost.

SUMMARY

The ability to diagnose and understand neurological conditions requires a good knowledge of normal neuroanatomy and the localization of neurological functions within the different parts of the central and peripheral nervous systems. Being able to determine which parts of the CNS and/or peripheral nervous system (PNS) must have been damaged to produce a particular defect and whether or not there is a single lesion, such as a tumour or vascular disruption, that could have caused a particular collection of defects, is fundamental to neurological diagnosis. Hence, learning the normal functional anatomy allows prediction of the functional pathology without much further effort. However, becoming familiar with the normal circuitry can take a little time and is best not left to the last minute.

A 29-year-old woman presents to her GP having lost 1 kg in weight despite a marked increase in her appetite. She has also noticed that she is sweating a great deal more than usual, even allowing for the warm summer weather. Some of her friends have remarked that she is uncharacteristically irritable and she has also been troubled by an increase in the frequency of her bowel motions from once a day to three times a day; there is no blood or mucus in her stool.

On examination the patient has a staring expression and shows exophthalmos. Lid retraction and lid lag are also present. The patient has a smooth, anterior midline neck mass around the level of the larynx that is symmetrical and moves upwards on swallowing. The patient has a fine resting tremor of her hands. Her pulse is 104 beats per minute and regular. Her reflexes are generally brisk, but the remainder of the examination is unremarkable.

Question 1

What is the diagnosis?

Answer 1

The patient is likely to have hyperthyroidism.

Although not definitive, the combination of weight loss and an increase in appetite, assuming there has not been a dramatic increase in physical activity, is very suggestive of hyperthyroidism. Malabsorption could also be considered as a cause of this combination, but the presence of steatorrhoea would be expected.

Many of the clinical features of hyperthyroidism can be predicted from knowledge of the normal functions of thyroxine. This principle applies to many other endocrine diseases.

Question 2

What are the causes of this condition?

Answer 2

- Graves' disease (see below)
- Solitary toxic nodule (an adenoma which secretes thyroxine autonomously)
- Toxic multinodular goitre
- Acute thyroiditis (surge of release of thyroxine from colloid due to inflammation)
- Exogenous thyroxine – iatrogenic or factitious
- Exogenous iodine
- Thyroid follicular cancer
- TSH-secreting tumour, including a pituitary adenoma (very rare)
- Hydatidiform mole (secretes high levels of beta-hCG, which has TSH-like actions)
- Amiodarone (contains iodine which can deregulate thyroid function).

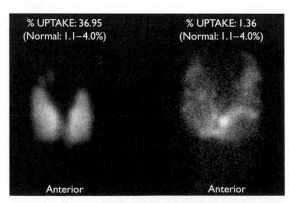

Figure 13.1 Nuclear medicine scan of the neck following intravenous injection of technetium-99 m pertechnate, which is taken up by the thyroid gland. (a) Smooth symmetrical enlargement of both lobes of the thyroid gland and markedly increased uptake of technetium-99 m pertechnate in a patient with hyperthyroidism related to Graves' disease. (b) Heterogeneous uptake in a patient with multinodular goitre.

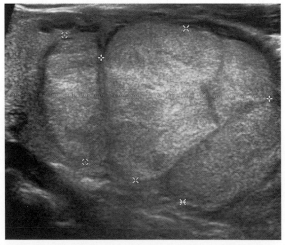

Figure 13.2 Ultrasound scan shows the presence of multiple nodules in the right lobe of the thyroid – multinodular goitre.

Question 3

What blood test would confirm the clinical diagnosis and what result would be expected?

Answer 3

Thyroid function tests which comprise thyroid-stimulating hormone (TSH) and thyroxine (T_4).

In hyperthyroidism, there would be expected to be an elevation of T_4 above the normal range and suppression of TSH below the normal range. The suppression of TSH reflects the fact that with the exception of the very rare TSH-secreting tumour, all of the other causes of hyper-thyroidism are independent of TSH. Therefore, TSH secretion by the pituitary is suppressed in response to detection of the elevated thyroxine levels in an attempt to restore normal levels (i.e. lower the level) of thyroxine.

Question 4

What is the neck mass?

Answer 4

The neck mass is the patient's enlarged thyroid gland. Thryoid masses are located in the anterior midline of the neck and move on swallowing, or with protrusion with the tongue.

Question 5

Patients with hyperthyroidism typically have a staring expression. What is the reason for this?

Answer 5

Hyperthyroidism produces sympathetic overactivation. Part of the innervation of the levator palpebrae superioris is from the sympathetic system. This results in retraction of the upper eyelid which in turn exposes more of the eye (characteristically sclera is seen between the edge of the eyelid and the iris, whereas this is not normally the case) and this generates a staring expression, as well as explaining the lid lag.

Question 6

Is it possible to predict the cause of the patient's hyperthyroidism in this case?

Answer 6

Yes. The presence of exophthalmos (abnormal protrusion of the eye anterior beyond the socket) is not due simply to the retraction of the upper eyelid that is common to all causes of hyperthyroidism, but instead reflects changes in the orbital soft tissues that are part of Graves' disease in particular. (While proptosis and exophthalmos are some-times used synonymously, some assert that exophthalmos implies Graves' disease specifically as the cause.) This exophthalmos can contribute to the staring expression.

In addition, the smooth and symmetrical enlarge-ment of the thyroid gland makes a multinodular goitre or a solitary adenoma, which are the two next most common causes of hyperthyroidism, less likely.

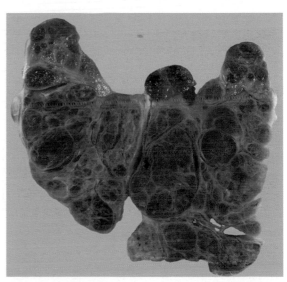

Figure 13.4 Multinodular goitre. Numerous dilated colloid-filled follicles give a glassy appearance to some of the nodules.

Effects of excess circulating thyroid hormone:

- Hot, sweaty, restless
- Exophthalmos, lid retraction, lid lag
- Goitre from enlarged thryroid
- Palpitations, arrhythmias, heart failure
- ↑appetite
- ↓weight
- Pre-tibial myxoedema

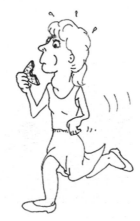

Figure 13.3 The typical features of hyperthyroidism.

Question 7

What is the cause of Graves' disease?

Answer 7

Graves' disease is an autoimmune condition in which circulating autoantibodies cross-react with the TSH receptor of the thyroid follicular epithelium causing aberrant activation of the receptor.

Question 8

What causes the exophthalmos?

Answer 8

As well as the effects on the TSH receptor, Graves' disease also features an autoimmune reaction against the soft tissues of the orbit. This produces inflammation with oedema and swelling, thereby forcing the orbital contents forwards.

Question 9

What complications can result from the ocular effects of Graves' disease?

Answer 9

In some instances, ocular Graves' disease can be severe. The eyelids cannot be closed properly, leading to drying of the cornea and corneal ulceration, scarring, opacification and visual loss. The lacrimal gland may be extruded, hampering tear production and worsening the problems associated with incomplete lid closure. Palsy of one or more of the extraocular muscles can develop. In extreme cases, Graves' ophthalmopathy can cause blindness.

Question 10

Given the basic pathological process that underlies Graves' disease, what macroscopic and microscopic changes would be expected in the thyroid gland?

Answer 10

The thyroid gland is being subjected to constant stimulation that mimics the effects of its natural trophic hormone. The response is one of hyperplasia. The autoantibody is systemic and exerts its effects to equal extent throughout the entire thyroid gland, so the hyperplasia is typically both diffuse and symmetrical. Hence, the thyroid gland is macroscopically enlarged in a symmetrical, generalized fashion.

Microscopically, the thyroid gland contains numerous follicles. As the follicular epithelial cells are being driven to produce large quantities of thyroxine, there is constant consumption of colloid at high levels. Thus the follicles tend to contain little colloid and may have scalloped borders as the epithelial cells attempt to increase the surface area available for colloid access.

The thyroid gland contains a lymphocytic infiltrate which is a manifestation of the underlying autoimmune process that is directed against the thyroid epithelium.

The thyroid gland often has an increased vascularity in Graves' disease which would be expected given the need for the follicles to secrete thyroxine into an attendant vasculature. This increase in vascularity is an important consideration if surgery is contemplated.

Question 11

Is hyperthyroidism more common in males or females?

Answer 11

Hyperthyroidism is considerably more common in women by a factor of around 5. This female predominance is a frequent finding in many autoimmune conditions (for example Hashimoto's thyroiditis, primary biliary cirrhosis, systemic lupus erythematosus).

CASE 14

HAEMATURIA CLINIC
A Sarah McKenzie Case

The tedium of Professor Paul's self-indulgent, rambling discourses had been a little softened for Sarah McKenzie by the passage of five months since she was last subjected to them. Now she found herself in the urology outpatient clinic, in the company of Mr Richard Shah, who was well liked among the students for his ability to impart useful knowledge.

'Right, this next patient has been referred by his GP because he has haematuria,' Mr Shah advised Sarah. 'That information alone should be enough to set off a chain of thoughts in your head. These will centre around knowing what the causes of haematuria could be and the associated anatomy, physiology and basic pathology. So, where could the haematuria be coming from?'

Sarah reckoned she was able to answer this question and worked through the urinary tract in her head. 'Well, it could be from the kidney, ureter, bladder or urethra.'

Mr Shah nodded, 'That's good. Is there anywhere else you should consider? How else might blood get into the urine, even if it wasn't originally from the urinary tract? This is probably more relevant in women.'

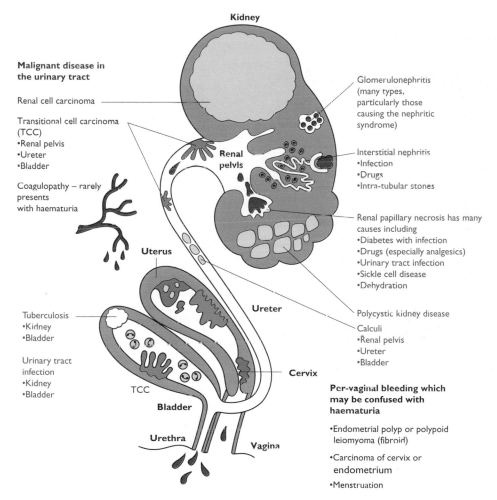

Figure 14.1 Causes of haematuria. Frank haematuria is seen with lower urinary tract lesions (e.g. urinary infection, bladder tumour or lower ureteric or bladder calculi). Bleeding from the higher reaches of the urinary tract will often appear 'smoky' due to altered blood. In these cases bleeding is occult and only detectable on urine testing (e.g. with a dipstick).

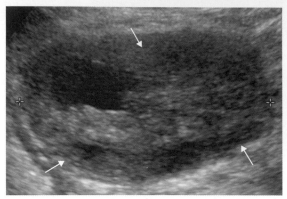

Figure 14.2 Transverse ultrasound image through the bladder showing a transitional cell carcinoma infiltrating virtually the entire bladder (arrows).

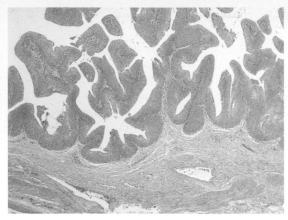

Figure 14.3 Low-power microscope image showing the papillary nature of transitional cell carcinoma of bladder. The tumour has not invaded the deeper layers of the bladder wall.

With the last hint, Sarah was able to grasp the point of Mr Shah's question. 'I suppose you could have contamination from menstrual blood.'

'Exactly. And perhaps as importantly, PV blood that is from abnormal bleeding in the female genital tract. Every now and then, when you're trying to find out why a particular person has haematuria, you might have to have a look around elsewhere if the urinary tract draws a blank.'

Question 1

What organs could be the source of haematuria?

Answer 1

- Kidney
- Ureter
- Bladder
- Urethra
- Contamination from the female genital tract.

'The next question,' went on Mr Shah, 'is how can these organs come to lose blood into the urinary tract? What sort of thing must be going on?'

'Some sort of damage,' suggested Sarah.

'Basically, yes. Something which damages the mucosa of any of the lining organs could cause bleeding. So what does that give us?'

'Tumours,' replied Sarah.

'Tumours are always a good one for bleeding from any orifice,' agreed Mr Shah, 'and that's where a lot of our work is focused. You can always supplement that answer with the division into benign and malignant, then malignant into primary and secondary. What are the main tumours in the urinary tract?'

'Transitional cell carcinomas?' offered Sarah.

'Correct, for the urothelium, but what about the kidney other than the renal pelvis.'

'Oh, renal cell carcinoma.'

'Yes. There are also benign renal tumours, but carcinoma is the most important. Moving away from tumours, what else could be going on?'

'Erm, UTI.'

'Good. And? What might be rattling around?'

'Stones!'

'Calculi, yes. Ureteric calculi can be very painful. Coming back to the kidney, there's an important group of conditions that cause haematuria.'

'I'm sorry, I can't think of them,' apologized Sarah.

'Well, where does the formation of urine first start?'

Sarah pondered her histology and physiology. 'The glomerulus. Glomerulonephritis.'

'Yes. They're very important. Left unchecked, some of them can wreck a kidney very rapidly. You can bracket interstitial nephritis and renal papillary necrosis with glomerulonephritis for the purposes of remembering your list. Don't forget TB either.'

'What about coagulopathies?' asked Sarah.

'That's a good point. A coagulopathy can exacerbate the blood loss from any existing injury, but in the absence of any damage, it shouldn't cause you to bleed spontaneously if absolutely everything is intact. The thing is, there are probably lots of very tiny microvascular breaches in the endothelium happening in various places across the body that normally are sealed without any fuss. If you have a really bad coagulopathy, these might start to become a problem.'

Question 2

What are the causes of haematuria?

Answer 2

- Glomerulonephritis (numerous causes)
- Interstitial renal disease (assorted causes)
- Renal papillary necrosis (various causes)
- Renal cell carcinoma
- Renal pelvis transitional cell carcinoma
- Transitional cell carcinoma of the ureter, bladder or urethra
- Other neoplasms of the bladder, ureter and urethra
- Urinary tract infection
- Tuberculosis
- Calculi
- Exacerbation by coagulopathies.

'We still haven't seen the patient yet,' noted Mr Shah, 'but things are already taking shape in our mind. The history and examination may well help to give us an idea of the likelihood of all these possibilities and help to guide us, but from what we know at present, what investigations seem to be on the cards?'

'I guess you'd do a full blood count to check the platelets and make sure the blood loss hadn't been going on long enough to cause anaemia. Check the coagulation and the U+Es.'

Mr Shah nodded, although seemed fairly neutral. 'Yes, that's all important, but as well as setting the background, what are you going to want to do that's more specific? The patient will be giving a urine sample for dipsticking, what else can you do with it?'

'Cytology? Twenty-four-hour urinary protein?'

'Cytology definitely. The urinary protein only if glomerular disease is particularly suspected. Cytology may well give you a diagnosis of a transitional cell carcinoma. All you have to do then is find out where it is, which gives you a clue for the other investigations.'

'Imaging,' said Sarah, 'ultrasound and CT.'

'Ultrasound is very useful. CT under some circumstances. Plain X-rays for stones. Another form of imaging, direct this time.'

'Cystoscopy,' offered Sarah, feeling that she was becoming comfortable with the topic.

'Yes. Have a look into the bladder and biopsy what's there.'

Question 3

What investigations might be relevant in haematuria?

Answer 3

The array of investigations will need to be tailored for each individual patient, especially if glomerular disease is suspected rather than a problem lower down the urinary tract, but urine cytology, imaging of the entire renal tract and cystoscopy are the cornerstones in the pursuit of a neoplastic cause.

Mr Shah brought the patient into the clinic room. The history and examination did not reveal any systemic symptoms and the blood tests that the GP had already arranged indicated that the patient had normal renal function. A dipstick was negative for protein. Mr Shah arranged a series of investigations along the lines he had discussed with Sarah.

Two weeks later, Sarah attended Mr Shah's cystoscopy list where the gentleman from the clinic was one of the patients. The cystoscopy revealed a small, papillary tumour on the trigone of the bladder. Mr Shah performed a transurethral resection of the tumour and told Sarah that they would aim to discuss the results at a forthcoming MDT (multi-disciplinary team) meeting.

At the MDT, the histopathology opinion was that the tumour was a pTa papillary transitional cell carcinoma. Mr Shah discussed the patient with Sarah after the meeting.

'What are transitional cell carcinomas, Sarah?' sought Mr Shah while other people were milling around trying to grab whatever remaining components of the free food they could.

'They're malignant tumours of the transitional cell mucosa. Some people call it the urothelium.'

'And what does pTa mean?'

'I'm not that sure. T is the stage of the primary tumour and the p in front means that's the pathologist's assessment of the stage, but I haven't come across the a.'

Mr Shah nodded. 'Not all organs have an 'a' stage. In the bladder, pTa tumours have a very good prognosis because they form a papillary outgrowth on the surface, but don't invade the bladder as such, so they don't have the chance to spread anywhere. Do you know any risk factors?'

Sarah recalled reading this. 'Smoking is one. The highest increased risk is from aniline dyes. I think they're used in the rubber and cable industries, so they're not a common risk factor, but they are very powerful ones.'

'That's the main thing, so always make sure to get an occupational history from the patient. Issues like compensation might apply. Now, in this gentleman's case, he presented with haematuria. How else could a transitional cell carcinoma present?'

Haematuria had always seemed the main clinical feature to Sarah, so she had to think. 'Pain? I guess, if they're in the ureter or urethra or the ureteric orifice, they could cause obstruction. Could they irritate the bladder and give things like urgency?'

'They're all possible. Don't forget that some people will be unfortunate enough to present with the features of distant metastases, or just a palpable primary mass. But haematuria is the main presenting complaint.'

Realizing that Sarah had to attend a pharmacology lecture, Mr Shah ended the discussion but suggested that she pop up to the ward later to see how the patient was doing post-operatively.

A 49-year-old woman seeks help from her GP because she has been bothered by shortness of breath on exertion for the past five months, together with a dry cough. She normally walks up the four flights of stairs to her office at work but she now becomes too short of breath after one. Nobody else in her office has noticed breathing problems. She has no other symptoms. Her previous medical history is unremarkable. She has no pets or hobbies that involve animals or chemicals. She has no history of exposure to asbestos. Her family history is unremarkable.

On examination, her trachea is central but there is symmetrically decreased expansion bilaterally. The percussion note is normal. Bilateral basal fine crackles are heard throughout both lung fields. Examination of the heart and abdomen is unremarkable.

The GP organizes a referral to the local respiratory medicine outpatient clinic where some further investigations are arranged.

Investigations

Full blood count	Normal
Urea and electrolytes (U+E)	Normal
Autoantibody screen	Negative
Arterial blood gases (on air)	
pH	7.42
pO_2	9.1 kPa
pCO_2	4.9 kPa
HCO_3^-	20 mmol/L
Lung function tests	
PEFR	Normal for age
FEV	Reduced
FVC	Reduced
FEV_1/FVC	Normal
Chest X-ray	See Figure 15.1

Question 1

What pattern of lung disease is revealed by the patient's lung function tests?

Answer 1

The patient has a restrictive pattern of disease.

Question 2

What pathological process is occurring in the lungs to produce this functional pattern?

Answer 2

Interstitial fibrosis.

Question 3

What are the causes of pulmonary fibrosis?

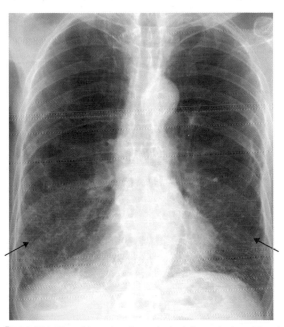

Figure 15.1 Chest X-ray showing reticular infiltrate in the mid and lower zones of both lungs (arrows), a feature of idiopathic pulmonary fibrosis.

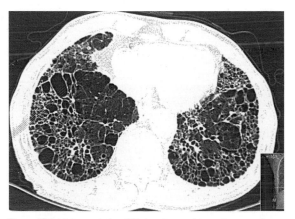

Figure 15.2 High-resolution CT showing endstage changes of idiopathic pulmonary fibrosis with honeycombing (arrowhead) and diffuse thickening of the peripheral interstitium/septa representing fibrosis (arrows).

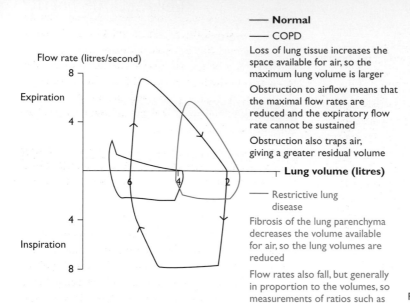

Flow rate (litres/second)

8

Expiration

4

Lung volume (litres)

6   4   2

4

Inspiration

8

—— **Normal**

—— COPD

Loss of lung tissue increases the space available for air, so the maximum lung volume is larger

Obstruction to airflow means that the maximal flow rates are reduced and the expiratory flow rate cannot be sustained

Obstruction also traps air, giving a greater residual volume

—— Restrictive lung disease

Fibrosis of the lung parenchyma decreases the volume available for air, so the lung volumes are reduced

Flow rates also fall, but generally in proportion to the volumes, so measurements of ratios such as FEV_1/FVC are preserved, wheras in COPD they are reduced

Figure 15.3 Basic flow volume loops for normal, obstructive disease and restrictive disease.

Answer 3

- Cryptogenic fibrosing alveolitis
- Extrinsic allergic alveolitis
- Industrial lung disease, e.g. asbestos, silicosis, berylliosis, coal dust
- Scleroderma
- Systemic lupus erythematosus
- Rheumatoid arthritis
- Radiation
- Drugs, e.g. bleomycin, amiodarone, gold
- Renal tubular acidosis
- Vasculitis can also cause a restrictive pattern of disease
- Tuberculosis is also associated with fibrosis, but is not usually diffuse.

Question 4

No underlying cause is found for the patient's disease and a working diagnosis of cryptogenic fibrosing alveolitis (CFA) (also known as idiopathic pulmonary fibrosis) is made. However, a lung biopsy is performed in order to support the diagnosis and to determine the subtype. The specimen is sent to the histopathology department with a request form that supplies the following information '?Fibrosis.' Is this adequate information?

Answer 4

No. The information is woefully inadequate. The request form should include a summary of the history and examination, blood tests, lung function tests and imaging. Without much more effort, the form could have been completed as:

Previously fit and well. 5/12 Hx SOBOE 1 flight of stairs. Non-smoker, no pets, dust or asbestos exposure. Widespread fine crackles. FBC, autoAb normal. Hypoxia on arterial blood gases. Restrictive pattern on lung function tests. CXR and CT – fibrosis, favour cryptogenic fibrosing alveolitis.

This information allows the pathologist to integrate the data with the histopathological findings and substantially increases the likelihood that they will be able to give a precise diagnosis, rather than just placing the changes in a general descriptive category.

Question 5

The lung biopsy confirms the presence of fibrosis, does not find any underlying cause and determines that the pattern of changes is that of usual interstitial pneumonia (UIP). What pathological process gives rise to the fibrosis?

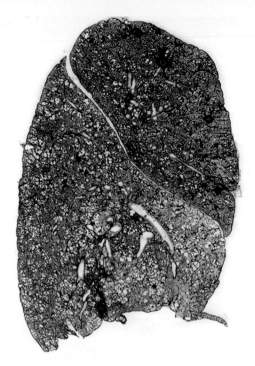

Figure 15.4 Wholemount slice of lung discussed in question 10.

Crackles occur when stiff airways distend. Airways can become stiff if their walls are thickened with collagen, or oedema (for example in cardiac failure).

Thickening of the alveolar septa increases the distance across which gases must diffuse. This impairs gas transfer between the blood and the air. At a certain point, this impairment will be sufficient to produce abnormalities in the blood gases.

Question 7

Why does this patient have hypoxia but not hypercapnia?

Answer 7

By virtue of its higher relative molecular mass, carbon dioxide has a greater diffusing capacity than oxygen. Therefore, it takes a greater degree of thickening of the alveolar septa to impair carbon dioxide exchange to the point at which hypercapnia develops. This greater degree of thickening occurs later in the disease than that at which oxygen exchange becomes compromised.

Question 8

The patient is placed on corticosteroids, although as is characteristically the case with the UIP variant of CFA, the response is poor. A year later, she is seen for her regular follow-up appointment. On examination, she is plethoric, her JVP (jugular venous pressure) is raised to 3 cm above the suprasternal notch, she has pitting oedema to the mid calf bilaterally, smooth hepatomegaly and a right parasternal heave. What has happened and why?

Answer 8

The patient has developed right heart failure. This is secondary to pulmonary hypertension, which in itself is secondary to her progressive lung disease. Most chronic lung diseases have the capacity to cause pulmonary hypertension. This is likely to reflect changes in pulmonary vascular tone that are secondary to changes in aeration and oxygen diffusion in the lung. It is a normal physiological response of the pulmonary vascular tree to shunt blood away from poorly ventilated volumes of the lung by vasoconstriction.

The pulmonary hypertension places a strain on the right heart, which has limited hypertrophic capacity. Ultimately, the elevated afterload exceeds the capacity of the right ventricle and the ventricle fails, with transmission of the pressure back through the systemic venous circulation.

Answer 5

The precise trigger that initiates events in CFA is not known. However, the process is one of chronic inflammation. The unknown stimulus damages the alveolar lining cells (type 1 pneumocytes) and capillary endothelial cells. Lymphocytes enter the interstitium of the lung. The cytokines released as part of the chronic inflammatory response stimulate the proliferation and activation of fibroblasts. The fibroblasts in turn secrete collagen.

Question 6

How does this pathological process produce the clinical picture?

Answer 6

The fibrosis thickens and stiffens the airways. This reduces their elasticity and compliance. As a consequence, the expansibility of the lungs is reduced and the lung volumes are decreased. Unlike obstructive diseases (such as chronic obstructive pulmonary disease, COPD), the reduction in volumes is proportionate and the FEV_1/FVC parameter, which is a ratio, is preserved.

Question 9

What could this patient's full blood count show?

Answer 9

The patient could have secondary polycythaemia. Chronic hypoxia is a stimulus for erythropoietin release. If less oxygen is available to the blood, increasing the density of erythrocytes will improve the ability of the blood to bind that oxygen which is available. However, once the haematocrit becomes too high, blood viscosity rises and there is a risk of thrombosis.

Question 10

Despite optimal treatment, the patient dies two years after diagnosis. Her relatives agree to a post mortem. Figure 15.4 shows a lung which could have come from this patient. What change is present?

Answer 10

The lung displays the 'honeycomb' pattern. This is the end-stage appearance in fibrosing lung diseases. The fibrosis reaches such a degree that it distorts the airways and pulls them into this honeycomb network.

A 31-year-old man undergoes a chest X-ray as part of the investigation of a dry cough that he has had for three months. The chest X-ray reveals bilateral hilar lymphadenopathy. A mediastinoscopic biopsy is obtained and the histopathology report includes the following:

> *The lymph node demonstrates numerous non-caseating granulomas that include multinucleate giant cells. Occasional asteroid bodies are seen. Special stains are negative for acid-fast bacilli and fungi. No malignancy is identified.*
>
> *Conclusion: Mediastinal lymph node: non-caseating granulomas.*

Question 1

What is a granuloma?

Answer 1

A granuloma is a collection of activated macrophages and usually forms in response to an antigen that is difficult to phagocytose by other means (see also Case 8: Abdominal pain and weight loss (p. 26), and Case 10: The ancient mimic (p. 34)).

Question 2

What is caseation?

Answer 2

Caseation is a particular form of necrosis that macroscopically resembles cheese and is very strongly associated with tuberculosis.

Question 3

What are acid-fast bacilli?

Answer 3

Acid-fast bacilli, such as mycobacteria, are difficult to stain with the usual methods (e.g. the Gram stain), so the Ziehl–Neelsen (ZN) stain is used. The term acid-fast bacilli is used synonymously with mycobacteria.

Question 4

Do the negative special stains exclude infection with the corresponding organisms?

Answer 4

No. The stains are performed on a section that is only a sample of the entire specimen and are also subject to technical and interpretative variables.

Question 5

Does the absence of caseation exclude tuberculosis?

Answer 5

No. Tuberculosis (TB) is not always accompanied by caseation, nor do necrotic granulomas always imply TB.

Question 6

What conditions can produce granulomas (not necessarily mediastinal)?

Answer 6

- Tuberculosis
- Atypical mycobacteria
- Fungal infection
- Parasitic infection
- Syphilis
- Sarcoidosis
- Wegener's granulomatosis
- Berylliosis
- Foreign body
- Crohn's disease
- Primary biliary cirrhosis
- Hodgkin's lymphoma
- As part of the response to other malignancies.

This list should not be considered to be exhaustive.

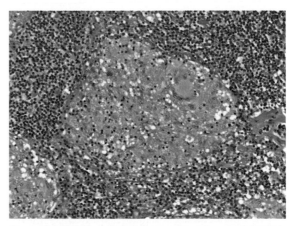

Figure 16.1 Microscope image of a granuloma (arrowed) located in a background of small lymphocytes. Unlike tuberculosis, where granulomas coalesce to form large masses with central necrosis, sarcoid granulomas are usually discrete from one another and do not show caseation necrosis.

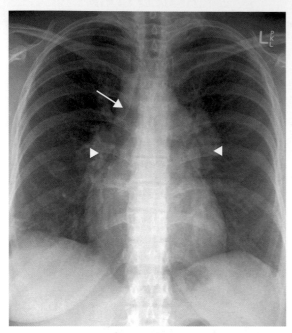

Figure 16.2 Chest X-ray showing bilateral hilar adenopathy (arrowheads) and right paratracheal adenopathy (arrow) in a 30-year-old woman with sarcoidosis.

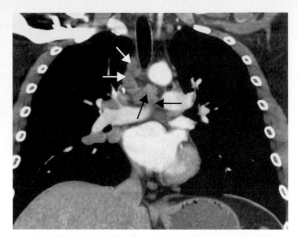

Figure 16.3 Coronal CT showing clusters of mediastinal and hilar lymph nodes (arrows) in the same patient as in Figure 16.2.

Question 7

The clinical history and examination are crucial for resolving the differential diagnosis of this man's mediastinal granulomatous lymphadenopathy. However, what other investigations should be performed and why?

Answer 7

As well as sending the lymph node for histopathology, material should be dispatched to microbiology. In addition to staining for the organism upon the initial receipt of the specimen, the microbiology department can culture the specimen in order to amplify the number of organisms that are present and thereby increase the likelihood that they will be detected. The properties of the organism that are manifested in culture will also help to identify it. Note that different organisms, such as mycobacteria and fungi, require specific culture media and the request form that accompanies the specimen should alert the pathology departments to the various possibilities in order that the specimen can be handled optimally. A greater array of techniques for subtyping an organism are available to microbiologists than histopathologists.

Optimal treatment of an infection requires not just identifying the causative organism but determining to which antibiotics that organism is sensitive and to which it is resistant. This cannot be accomplished by the histopathology department with fixed material and is the province of microbiology, using the organisms that they have grown from culture.

Approximately 70 per cent of patients with sarcoidosis have an elevated serum angiotensin-converting enzyme (ACE) level and this can be readily measured.

Assorted autoantibodies can be measured to evaluate the possibility of vasculitis.

Question 8

In this patient, the lymph node culture was negative, his serum ACE level was increased, an autoantibody screen was negative and he also had a history of uveitis and skin rashes. A diagnosis of sarcoidosis was made. What is sarcoidosis?

Answer 8

Sarcoidosis is a chronic, multi-system disorder of uncertain aetiology that is characterized by the presence of non-caseating granulomas that may develop in various organs. A vasculitic component may also be present. Sarcoidosis typically affects the lungs and mediastinal lymph nodes. The skin, eye and parotid gland are other characteristic sites.

Question 9

The patient's blood calcium level was also measured. Why?

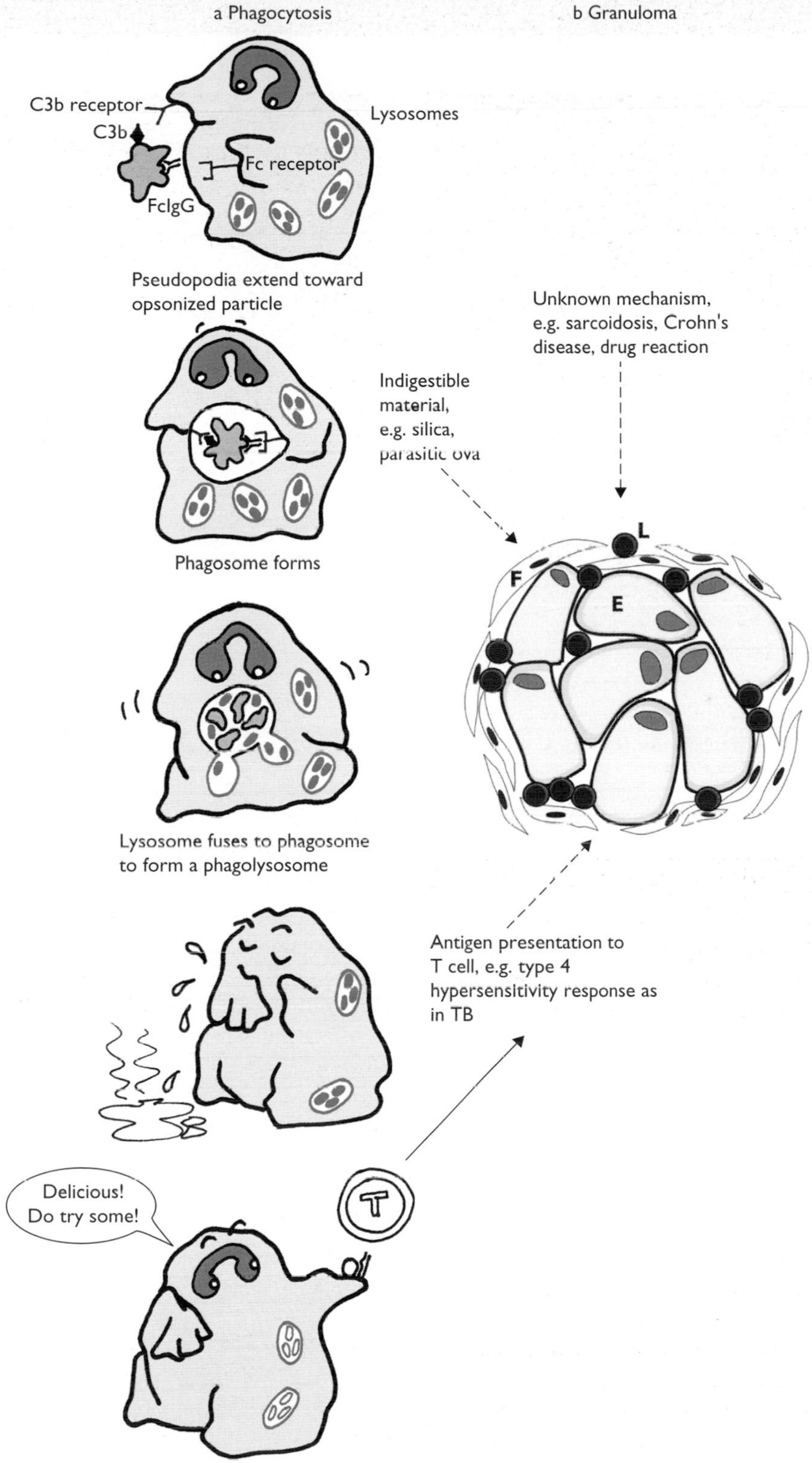

Figure 16.4 Causes of granuloma formation. (a) Normal stages of phagocytosis by macrophages. (b) Granulomas are collections of epithelioid giant cells formed in a variety of circumstances. In tuberculosis, the mycobacterium prevents the phagolysosome forming and a type 4 hypersensitivity response drives the macrophages to alter their phenotype to become epithelioid cells and cluster together as granulomas. E, epithelioid cells; F, fibroblasts; L, lymphocytes.

Answer 9

Approximately 10 per cent of patients with sarcoidosis have hypercalcaemia. This is due to the presence of the 1-alpha-vitamin D hydroxylase enzyme within the macrophages of the sarcoidal granulomas. These macrophages mediate an inappropriate activation of vitamin D and hypercalcaemia can result. It is said that this process is a property of all granulomatous conditions, but is only typically described in sarcoidosis.

A 27-year-old woman presents to her GP with a two-month history of night sweats and a two-week history of a low-grade fever. She has previously been fit and well and is taking no medication other than the oral contraceptive pill. She has not noticed any other symptoms, such as a cough, dysuria or earache, which could explain her night sweats and pyrexia.

Question 1

Does the patient's fever classify as a pyrexia of unknown origin?

Answer 1

Pyrexia of unknown origin (PUO) is a fever that persists for at least three weeks in the absence of an ascertained cause. In the case of this patient, the three-week criterion has not yet been reached. It could also be argued that attempts to determine the cause of the fever have yet to be commenced.

The term PUO is not a diagnosis, in the same way that neither dysphagia nor haemoptysis are. Instead, it is a category of presentation and clinical features which focuses and guides investigation and the process of diagnosis. Such labels are useful because they encapsulate causes and concepts, which then allow a methodological approach.

Question 2

What are the causes of fever, with particular regard to a PUO?

Answer 2

Fever is an elevation of the body's temperature and is usually due to inflammatory mediators acting on the hypothalamus to adjust the regulation of body temperature to a higher level. There are various conditions that can produce this effect:

- Infection (TB is especially important in PUO, as are unusual infections)
- Neoplasia
- Vasculitis
- Chronic autoimmune disease, especially collagen vascular diseases (systemic lupus erythematosus, rheumatoid arthritis, scleroderma)
- Hyperthyroidism
- Rare intracranial tumours – these operate by damaging the hypothalamus
- Inherited disorders of autonomic function (very rare).

Despite not meeting the defining criteria for having a PUO, this patient nevertheless has a history that merits investigation. While the fever may not yet have endured for three weeks, she has no other symptoms which clearly account for it and it is accompanied by night sweats which predate it and are also unexplained.

On examination, the GP finds several small masses that are situated laterally in both sides of the neck. The masses are subcutaneous, rubbery, non-tender and are up to 20 mm in size.

Question 3

What are the masses?

Answer 3

The masses are lymph nodes. Although there are assorted causes of lumps in the neck, lymph nodes are the only ones that plausibly fit this description. However, the importance in real life of being able to feel the masses for yourself and comparing that with the experience of the properties of previous lymph nodes should not be underestimated.

Question 4

In more general terms, what lumps can be found in the neck?

Answer 4

- Thyroid – central, anterior, moves on swallowing, may be associated with symptoms of thryoid dysfunction
- Thyroglossal cyst – also central, anterior and moves on protusion of the tongue, but situated more superiorly than the thyroid
- Branchial cyst – a developmental remnant, found laterally, typically in the upper part of the neck
- Lymph nodes – located laterally, various consistencies
- Skin tumours.

Question 5

The GP refers the patient to the local head and neck department where she is seen a week after her initial presentation. What investigation that is immediately available in the outpatient department is most likely to yield the diagnosis?

Answer 5

Fine needle aspiration (FNA) of one or more of the lymph nodes. FNA is a cytological technique in which a needle is introduced into a target mass and material is aspirated into the needle by use of suction applied by a syringe attached to the needle (some operators, under some conditions, find the use of the capillary action to draw material into the needle gives good samples, but aspiration is employed in most instances). The tissue obtained can either be smeared directly onto a slide for staining, or placed into a liquid medium. Centrifugation handling of the suspension of cells enables multiple preparations to be made from one of these liquid samples.

Question 6

What are the advantages of FNA compared with a histological biopsy?

Answer 6

FNA can be performed quickly, without the need for anaesthetic and requires little specialist equipment. The tissue does not need to be fixed in the same way as histology and this can speed things up by a day or so. Part of the sample can also be sent to microbiology without having been rendered of limited to no use by fixation.

FNA tends to be well tolerated by the patient and has a very low risk of complications.

Question 7

What are the disadvantages of FNA compared with a histological biopsy?

Answer 7

The FNA sample captures very little of the architecture of the disease process. The little architecture which may be preserved tends to be only that of how clusters of cells configure themselves; information regarding larger formations, invasion and the relationship to the stroma is lost and this low-power information is often vital.

The quantity of tissue obtained by FNA is less than for a histological sample.

Unused material from an FNA cannot be stored indefinitely. By contrast, the paraffin-processed, formalin-fixed blocks generated in histology last for decades and can be returned to if needed.

Even with the limitations secondary to the lack of architectural information, FNA is a valuable technique that in skilled hands (both in obtaining a good sample and interpreting it) can frequently yield a firm diagnosis.

Question 8

The patient is seen with the findings of the FNA in the outpatient department in a follow-up appointment shortly afterwards. The ENT consultant explains that the patient has a disease called lymphoma. What is lymphoma and how is it classified?

Answer 8

Lymphoma is a malignant tumour of lymphocytes.

The main division in the classification of lymphoma is into Hodgkin's lymphoma and non-Hodgkin's lymphoma (NHL). Categorization of NHL has been notoriously complicated over the years and the finer points have in the past rested upon the morphology of the cells. The relatively recent World Health Organization (WHO) classification adopts an approach which reflects the presumptive cell of origin and incorporates morphological, immunohistochemical and sometimes genetic parameters.

Question 9

What is the importance of precise classification of lymphomas?

Answer 9

Different lymphomas have different behaviour, prognoses and sensitivity to particularly chemotherapy

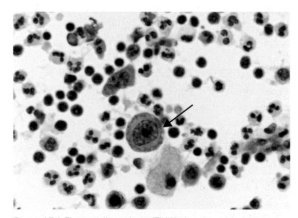

Figure 17.1 Fine needle aspirate (FNA) showing a Hodgkin–Reed–Sternberg (HRS) cell in a background of mixed inflammatory cells.

regimens so require different treatments. If they were all lumped together, treatment would not be as effective and morbidity and mortality would be higher. One of the advantages of the WHO system is that the different entities are of prognostic significance.

Even with the WHO scheme, the classification of lymphomas is detailed and too lengthy to discuss in this book. The important principles are the division into Hodgkin's and non-Hodgkin's lymphoma, with the subdivision of NHL into B cell lymphomas and T cell lymphomas. B cell lymphomas may be considered as low grade or high grade. Most T cell lymphomas behave in a high grade fashion. B cell NHL accounts for around 90 per cent of NHL.

Question 10

The patient's FNA contains cells similar to those shown in Figure 17.1. What is this cell?

Answer 10

The cell is a Hodgkin–Reed–Sternberg cell (HRS cell). HRS cells are characteristic of Hodgkin's lymphoma. The classical Reed–Sternberg cell is large and has a bilobed nucleus, in each lobe of which is a large, eosinophilic nucleolus. Other variants exist, including the mononuclear form shown in Figure 17.1, and the term 'HRS cell' provides a more encompassing designation for this broader group. HRS cells are derived from B cells.

Note the background of neutrophils and small lymphocytes in Figure 17.1. The small lymphocytes provide a useful scale against which to compare the size of the HRS cell. One of the curious features of Hodgkin's lymphoma is that the actual HRS cells comprise only a very small fraction of the cells in an affected lymph node yet are able to behave as a neoplastic disease. Most of the accompanying cells in Hodgkin's lymphoma are small lymphocytes with variable numbers of macrophages and neutrophils. The proportion of non-lymphocyte cells is greater in some subtypes. Eosinophils are often found and are a useful assisting feature.

Question 11

What is the significance of the patient's presenting symptoms?

Answer 11

The fever and night sweats are both termed 'B symptoms' in lymphoma. The other B symptom is unintentional weight loss of at least 10 per cent. B symptoms are included in the staging system: patients without B symptoms have an A suffix (Figure 17.2).

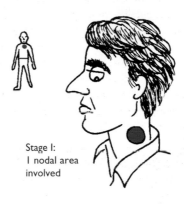

Stage I:
1 nodal area involved

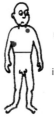

Stage II: ≥2 nodal areas on same side of diaphragm involved (no. of involved sites recorded)

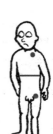

Stage III: nodal areas on each side of diaphragm:
III$_1$ upper abdomen,
III$_2$ lower abdomen

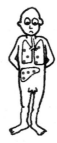

Stage IV:
visceral involvement

The spleen is part of the reticuloendothelial system. Splenic involvement does not carry the same staging implications as bone marrow or liver

Figure 17.2 Cotswold revision of the Ann Arbor staging system for Hodgkin's lymphoma. The presence of 'B symptoms' (e.g. fever, drenching night sweats, weight loss) adversely affects the prognosis and is included in the staging (e.g. stage IIA – no B symptoms; stage IIB – B symptoms present).

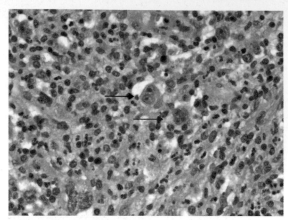

Figure 17.3 Paraffin section showing classical binuclear Reed–Sternberg cells in the centre of the image (black arrow). Just below and to the right is a Hodgkin–Reed–Sternberg (HRS) cell with a more complex nuclear configuration (red arrow). Note that the vast majority of cells in the field are not HRS cells but are instead small lymphocytes, macrophages, eosinophils and neutrophils.

Question 12

How is Hodgkin's lymphoma staged?

Answer 12

Like NHL, Hodgkin's lymphoma is staged by the Ann Arbor system (Figure 17.2). Since lymphoma primarily involves lymph nodes, and lymphocytes (benign and malignant) may circulate and home to particular nodal

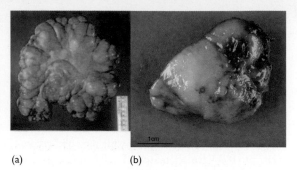

(a)   (b)

Figure 17.4 (a) Typical rubbery matted mass of lymph nodes seen in lymphoma. (b) A single node, sliced to show the bland, fleshy appearance of lymphoma. Hodgkin's lymphoma may appear slightly nodular, as seen here.

groups, it is not possible to use the TNM staging system. The Ann Arbor classification addresses the disease status in terms of the nodal groups involved and the presence or absence of extranodal disease.

The patient proceeds to have a lymph node excision biopsy. While FNA can accurately diagnose Hodgkin's lymphoma, histology is necessary to determine the subtype and to confirm the diagnosis as there can be rare morphological overlaps with some types of NHL. A bone marrow aspirate and trephine is undertaken at the same time as part of the staging.

A 51-year-old woman notices swelling of her right calf in the taxi ride home from the airport after a transatlantic flight. It is one o'clock in the morning and she is very tired and preoccupied with finally having the chance to lie down and go to bed, so does not pay close attention to her leg.

Shortly after waking up the following morning, she develops a sudden onset of shortness of breath that is associated with central chest pain. The pain has no radiation and is not associated with nausea or vomiting. The woman calls an ambulance and is taken to the accident and emergency department.

On arrival she is tachypnoeic, although is able to speak in short sentences and does not have central cyanosis. Her pulse is 108 beats per minute and regular. Her blood pressure is 110/70 mmHg. The apex beat is normal. The heart sounds are normal and there are no added sounds or murmurs. Examination of the lungs and abdomen is normal.

The patient's right calf is red, swollen and tender. The circumference of the calf is 5 cm greater than that of the left.

The ECG shows sinus tachycardia.

Investigations

Arterial blood gases (on room air)

pH	7.50
pO_2	9.1 kPa
pCO_2	3.5 kPa
HCO_3^-	19 mmol/L

Question 1

What is the diagnosis?

Answer 1

The patient has a pulmonary embolism (PE) secondary to a right lower limb deep vein thrombosis (DVT).

Question 2

What normal mechanisms exist to oppose coagulation and to remove thrombi?

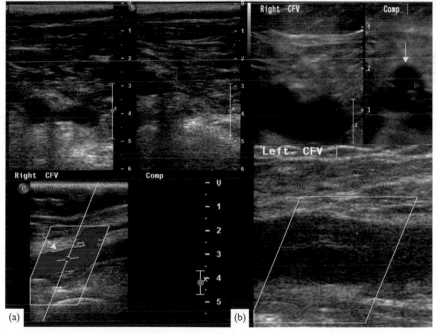

Figure 18.1 (a) Venous duplex ultrasound of the common femoral vein showing a normal right femoral vein which compresses with probe pressure (red arrow) and demonstrates colour flow filling the entire vessel (yellow arrow). (b) Venous duplex ultrasound is the investigation of choice for the detection of deep venous thrombosis (DVT). In an acute DVT, the vein fails to completely compress on probe pressure (yellow arrow), clot fills the lumen of the vein (red arrow) and there is no colour flow in the vein (box).

Answer 2

As well as possessing systems for generated thrombus, the body has both anti-thrombotic and fibrinolytic pathways.

Inappropriate activation of the thrombotic system can have catastrophic effects and therefore blood clotting must be closely regulated. As well as the control that is provided by the requirement for specific triggers to activate clotting, there are also pathways in place that actively oppose thrombosis. Under normal circumstances, a thrombus will only develop when the stimulus for its development exceeds the opposition provided by the normal background of the anti-thrombotic pathway.

Once a thrombus has developed, a system needs to be in place to remove the thrombus once it has served its purpose. This system is the fibrinolytic pathway. Therapeutic use is made of this pathway with drugs such as streptokinase and recombinant tissue plasminogen activator (rtPA or tPA).

Question 3

What factors would cause a patient to be hypercoaguable?

Answer 3

There are various conditions which can make a person more prone to thrombosis. Those which are particularly associated with a DVT are:

- immobility
- flight in a pressurized aircraft
- obstruction to the venous outflow.

However, there are numerous other factors that are more general and can be overlooked. These relate to the constituents of the blood and the coagulation system:

- dehydration
- protein C deficiency
- protein S deficiency
- factor V Leiden
- antiphospholipid syndrome
- polycythaemia
- thrombocytosis
- hyperviscosity (e.g. myeloma)
- paroxysmal nocturnal haemoglobinuria
- paraneoplastic syndromes
- vasculitis.

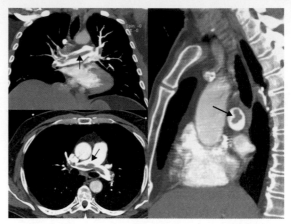

Figure 18.2 CT pulmonary angiography is the investigation of choice for detecting pulmonary embolism. The technique relies on a bolus of intravenous iodinated contrast given through a large cannula in a proximal arm vein with the scan being timed to start during maximal opacification of the pulmonary arterial tree. Note the saddle embolus (arrows) from a deep vein thrombosis of the leg lying across the bifurcation of the pulmonary outflow tract.

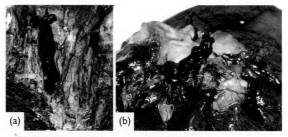

Figure 18.3 (a) Fresh thrombus within an opened popliteal vein and (b) a pulmonary embolus lying within the pulmonary artery at the hilum of the lung.

Question 4

Why is examination and imaging of the pelvis important?

Answer 4

Some lower limb DVTs are secondary to compression of the iliac vessels by a tumour mass within the pelvis. If this possibility is overlooked, an opportunity to diagnose a malignant neoplasm may be missed.

Question 5

What is an embolism in general and a pulmonary embolism in particular?

Answer 5

An embolus is a substance carried in the blood which lodges in and obstructs vessel(s) distant to the point of origin of the embolus. A pulmonary embolus is one which lodges in the pulmonary arterial system.

Question 6

What are the pathophysiological consequences of a pulmonary embolism (PE)?

Answer 6

A PE will result in a region of lung that is ventilated but not perfused. If this region is large enough, the volume of lung tissue lost for gas exchange will be sufficient to produce hypoxia.

The region of the lung that has suffered a reduction in blood flow will become ischaemic and may infarct (the dual supply from the bronchial arteries often prevents infarction). It will show a decrease in surfactant production within a few hours, leading to atelectasis in 12–15 hours.

The PE reduces the cross-sectional area of the pulmonary vasculature. However, as pulmonary blood flow remains the same, the total pulmonary vascular resistance against which the right ventricle must work increases. Nevertheless, approximately 50 per cent of the pulmonary bed must be lost before pulmonary

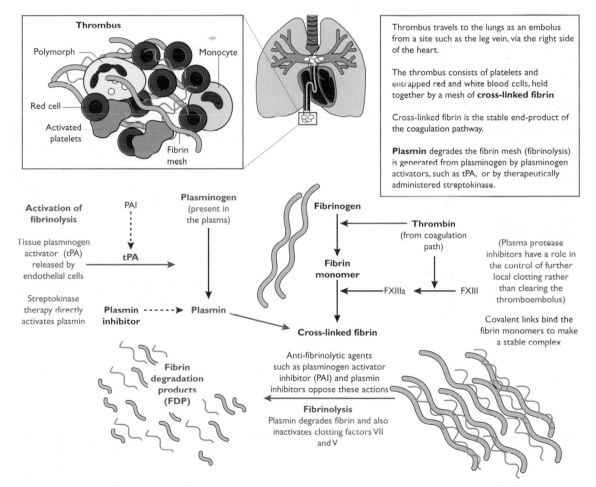

Figure 18.4 Thrombosis and thrombolysis exist in a dynamic equilibrium. Several anticoagulant mechanisms exist, including antithrombin, tissue factor plasma inhibitor, thrombomodulin and protein kinases C and S. Of importance once a thrombus has embolized is the body's fibrinolytic mechanisms, shown here. As fibrin is formed and cross-linked, plasminogen in the plasma is incorporated within the thrombus. Plasminogen activator is secreted by activated or damaged endothelial cells and forms plasmin, which lyses fibrin. Streptokinase and newer drugs with similar actions can also activate plasminogen.

hypertension ensues. If the increase in pulmonary resistance is great enough, strain will be placed upon the right side of the heart. Unlike the left ventricle, the right has a significantly limited inotropic capacity, particularly in the face of a sudden increase in afterload. If the PE is sufficiently large, right heart failure can occur; any pre-existing heart disease may lower the threshold at which this happens.

The largest types of PE, those that occlude the main pulmonary trunk, are fatal because they prevent any circulation through the pulmonary vasculature and stop blood from reaching the left side of the heart.

Question 7

Other than the tachypnoea, examination of this patient's lungs was normal. Is that to be expected?

Answer 7

Yes. Ventilation of the lungs is not disturbed and therefore parameters such as expansion, percussion and auscultation will be unaffected.

Question 8

What is the reason for the appearance of the right calf?

Answer 8

The DVT in the right lower limb hampers venous drainage of the limb. This results in congestion and accounts for the clinical features of being red, swollen and tender.

Question 9

In view of the pathophysiology of a pulmonary embolus, what features could be expected on examination of the heart (not necessarily in this case)?

Answer 9

The cardiac signs of a PE are variable and those that are dependent on right heart strain or failure only occur with larger emboli.

- Sinus tachycardia is relatively common and is an attempt to overcome the ventilation perfusion mismatch by increasing pulmonary blood flow.
- Atrial fibrillation can be caused by a PE and reflects acute dilatation of the right atrium secondary to an inability of the right ventricle to cope with the increased afterload. As a rule of thumb, any cause of dilatation of the atria can cause atrial fibrillation.
- Large PEs can produce hypotension by decreasing the venous return to the left side of the heart. In extreme cases, this takes the form of pulseless electrical activity.
- Significant right heart failure will elevate the jugular venous pressure (JVP).
- Forceful right ventricular contractions against the elevated pulmonary vascular resistance may be palpated as a right ventricular heave.

Question 10

What abnormalities are present in this patient's blood gases and what is the cause?

Answer 10

The patient has hypoxia and a respiratory alkalosis.

The hypoxia is due to a sufficiently large volume of lung tissue being prevented from taking part in gas transfer by the embolus. The hypoxia triggers hyperventilation and this results in a loss of carbon dioxide, leading to the alkalosis. Even though the loss of lung tissue is enough to produce hypoxia, the higher diffusing capacity of carbon dioxide means that adequate lung tissue remains to permit effective handling of carbon dioxide. However, with the largest PEs carbon dioxide transfer is also compromised and hypercapnoea occurs.

Malcolm Granger, aged 48, has just left hospital. He was hit by a car as he inebriatedly weaved his way home by bicycle from a rugby club dinner (he lost his licence for drink-driving a year ago). His injuries were mild, but he had hit his head and cracked his skull so he was kept in for observation. After a day the nurses noted that he was plucking agitatedly at his sheets and cringing from 'vultures' circling him. He was also sweating, with a tachycardia and rapid breathing. The registrar diagnosed delirium tremens, caused by acute alcohol withdrawal. Malcolm's claim at the time of admission was that he only 'drank socially'! Malcolm recovered with medication (diazepam, then clomethiazole, plus multivitamins) over the next two days. A psychiatric referral was made, but Malcolm denied an alcohol problem and discharged himself.

Question 1

What features of alcoholism can you recognize from this history?

Answer 1

- Drink-driving
- Accidents: road traffic, domestic
- Lack of awareness: denies alcohol problem

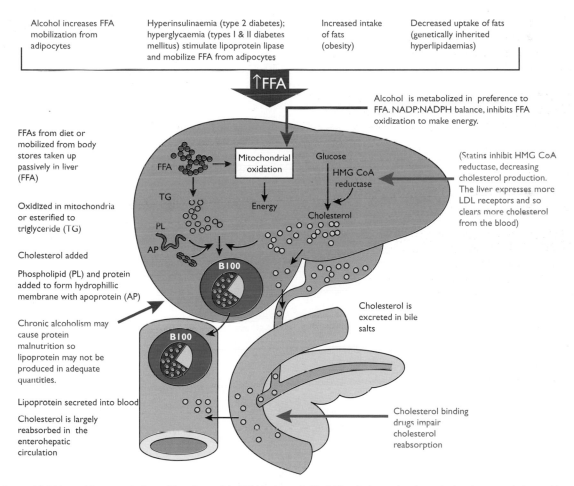

Figure 19.1 Normal liver metabolism of free fatty acids (FFA) is shown in black. The cholesterol pathway is also shown – cholesterol is also brought to the liver by high-density lipoproteins (HDL) and low-density lipoprotein (LDL). The points at which alcohol interacts are shown in red. The effects of drug treatment are shown in blue.

- Withdrawal symptoms: plucking bedclothes as if picking off ants is typical, also paranoid delusions.

Also may have:

- Dependence on alcohol early in the day, before meeting people
- Inability to cope at work
- Marital breakdown.

Question 2

Why treat with clomethiazole?

Answer 2

Clomethiazole stimulates increased release of GABA (gamma-aminobutyric acid), a neurotransmitter which induces sleepiness and controls anxiety. Some effects of alcohol are mediated through GABA receptors and rapid withdrawal may therefore cause problems. Clomethiazole also inhibits alcohol dehydrogenase.

One year later, Malcolm is rushed to intensive care in a weak, jaundiced and semi-comatose state. His breath is foul-smelling ('foetor hepaticus'). His sclerae are deep yellow and his liver is enlarged and tender. He is dirty and unshaven. He demonstrates asterixis. Investi-gations show that he is in fulminant liver failure.

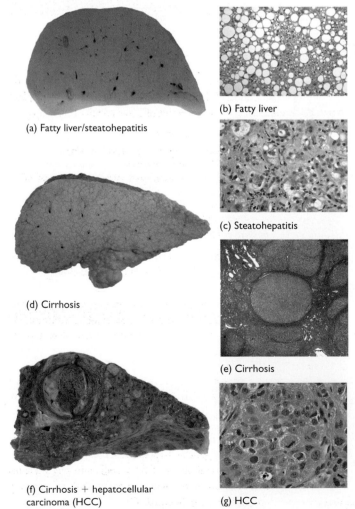

(a) Fatty liver/steatohepatitis

(b) Fatty liver

(c) Steatohepatitis

(d) Cirrhosis

(e) Cirrhosis

(f) Cirrhosis + hepatocellular carcinoma (HCC)

(g) HCC

Figure 19.2 Around 60% of chronic alcoholics will develop fatty liver (a,b); 40% will develop steatohepatitis, which looks similar macroscopically but shows inflammation and early fibrosis microscopically (c); 10–15% will develop cirrhosis, usually micronodular type (d,e); only 10% of people with cirrhosis will develop hepatocellular carcinoma (f,g).

Question 3

What are the clinical features of fulminant acute liver failure?

Answer 3

- Encephalopathy
  - grade I, mild confusion, euphoria or depression
  - grade II, drowsy and semi-comatose
  - grade III, stupor (marked confusion but rousable)
  - grade IV, coma (unrousable)
- Jaundice
- Bleeding tendency (often this is generalized oozing into the gastrointestinal tract)
- Asterixis ('liver flap'), a curious phenomenon which is demonstrated with the arms outstretched and the hands dorsiflexed – it reflects uraemia.

Question 4

What investigations would you perform and why?

Answer 4

1. Liver function tests (see Case 33 (p. 125) for further information):
   - metabolic function tests – transaminases (ALT and AST)
   - inducible liver enzymes – alkaline phosphatase, GGT
   - synthetic function tests – albumin, prothrombin time or INR
   - bilirubin.
2. Blood glucose: hypoglycaemia due to loss of gluconeogenesis carries a poorer prognosis.
3. Blood urea and creatinine levels: nitrosourea compounds are metabolized by the liver, so failure leads to high circulating blood levels. Interference with neurotransmitters causes confusion and coma. Nitrosourea compounds excreted in the breath cause foetor hepaticus.
4. Blood cultures, chest X-ray, urine culture: alcoholics are at increased risk of bacterial and fungal infection.
5. Ultrasound of the abdominal organs.
6. Liver biopsy: to demonstrate liver cell necrosis, inflammation and fibrosis.

Ultrasound scan shows a smoothly enlarged liver.

Investigations

(Indications for immediate referral for transplantation in bold.)

Bilirubin (>300)	437 μmol/L	(3–17 μmol/L)
ALT	1097 IU/L	(5–35 IU/L)
AST	997 IU/L	(5–35 IU/L)
ALP	443 IU/L	(30–150 IU/L)
Albumen	32 g/L	(35–48 g/L)
GGT	640 IU/L	(0–50 IU/L)
Urea	8.8 mmol/L	(2.5–6.7 mmol/L)
Creatinine (>300)	240 μmol/L	(70–170 μmol/L)
Glucose	3.3 mmol/L	(3.5–5 mmol/L (fasting))
pH (<7.3)	7.35	(7.4)
INR (>6.5)	6.3	(1.0)
PaO_2	11.4 kPa	(13.3 kPa)

The consultant hepatologist notes that the test results do not quite fulfil the criteria for referral to a liver transplant centre. He reads the result of a transjugular liver biopsy.

Summary of liver findings:

- *marked fatty change with Mallory's hyaline*
- *confluent hepatocyte necrosis*
- *acute inflammation and ballooning degeneration of hepatocytes*
- *cholestasis*
- *evidence of liver cell regeneration*
- *very mild fibrosis.*

Conclusion: appearances are those of florid steatohepatitis, compatible with an alcoholic aetiology.

Question 5

Discuss the factors that can generate a fatty liver, and its consequences.

Answer 5

Causes of fatty liver:

- Raised free fatty acids: alcohol excess, diabetes mellitus, obesity, genetic hyperlipidaemia
- Lowered metabolism of fatty acids and triglycerides (competition with drugs, e.g. alcohol or pathway interference, e.g. hepatitis C)

- Lowered excretion, e.g. due to lowered protein for synthesis of lipoprotein (chronic alcoholism, protein calorie malnutrition) or paralysis of the secretory apparatus (e.g. drugs of various types).

Consequences of fatty liver:

- Mechanically impaired blood flow in the hepatic sinusoids
- Oxidation of fat causes free radical formation, stimulating inflammation and fibrosis
- Hepatocyte insulin resistance (leads to type 2 diabetes mellitus)
- Fat can activate angiotensin, leading to hypertension.

Question 6

Compare fatty liver disease, steatohepatitis and acute liver failure.

Answer 6

Fatty liver shows fat with minimal inflammation and no fibrosis. This is reversible but about 50 per cent of patients later develop fibrosis. *Steatohepatitis* features fatty change, inflammation and ballooning of hepatocytes (a feature of toxic damage), often with fibrosis. Patients risk acute liver failure or advanced fibrosis/cirrhosis. *Acute liver failure* features massive hepatocyte necrosis due to a toxic insult such as alcohol, paracetamol overdose or acute viral (or other) hepatitis. The mortality in acute liver failure due to steatohepatitis is around 40 per cent. Recurrent attacks are common, each with 40 per cent risk.

After many weeks in hospital, Malcolm is ready to return home. He is warned that another episode could be fatal. If he continues to drink he will almost certainly develop cirrhosis.

Question 7

Compare the risk of severe liver disease due to alcohol with other aetiologies.

Answer 7

- Alcohol – 50 per cent steatohepatitis of whom 10–15 per cent have cirrhosis
- Non-alcoholic fatty liver disease – 40 per cent steatohepatitis of whom 5–10 per cent have cirrhosis
- Hepatitis B virus – 10 per cent chronic hepatitis of whom 10 per cent have cirrhosis

- Hepatitis C virus – 80 per cent chronic hepatitis of whom 10 per cent have cirrhosis.

Malcolm worries when 72-year-old Bill Barlow from his Alcoholics Anonymous group misses several meetings. Bill knew that his liver was cirrhotic but if he kept away from alcohol he should be all right for years. Bill found this impossible.

Question 8

Describe the microscopical features of cirrhosis.

Answer 8

Cirrhotic scarring is a diffuse process involving the entire liver. There is liver architectural destruction by nodules of regenerating hepatocytes separated by fibrous septa. If inflammation is present it indicates 'active' cirrhosis and further damage and scarring are likely.

Question 9

Is it true that someone with cirrhosis can remain well?

Answer 9

A patient with established cirrhosis but no inflammation may remain surprisingly well ('compensated cirrhosis'). Anything which causes inflammation or toxic damage to hepatocytes can precipitate liver failure.

Question 10

What are the main causes of cirrhosis?

Answer 10

Globally hepatitis B and C and alcohol are the main causes of cirrhosis. Common causes of cirrhosis in the UK are:

- Alcohol 60 per cent
- Hepatitis C: 5–10 per cent
- Hepatitis B: 5–10 per cent (viral hepatitis is the largest cause globally)
- Autoimmune hepatitis: 10 per cent
- Biliary disease: primary biliary cirrhosis, sclerosing cholangitis: 5–10 per cent
- Non-alcoholic steatohepatitis/metabolic syndrome: 5–10 per cent
- Metabolic causes, such as haemochromatosis or Wilson's disease are rare.

Malcolm learns that Bill has been rushed to hospital after vomiting blood. Bill is jaundiced, with ascites and spider naevi over his scrawny chest. Scans show a large nodule at the periphery of his cirrhotic liver and an enlarged spleen. In order to biopsy the peripherally located nodule, the ascitic fluid is drained and Bill is injected with vitamin K, to assist clotting factor synthesis by his residual liver tissue, and transfused with fresh frozen plasma at the time of biopsy.

Question 11

Which features of chronic liver disease does Bill display?

Answer 11

Features displayed by Bill:

- Jaundice
- Ascites: intraperitoneal transudate due to lowered plasma oncotic pressure (lowered serum albumin) and raised hydrostatic pressure from portal hypertension
- Portal hypertension and splenomegaly
- Nutritional problems (shoulder girdle wasting is typical)
- Coagulation problems
- Spider naevi (capillaries radiating from a central vessel, blanching on pressure) reflect high oestrogen levels. In cirrhosis and hepatocellular carcinoma numerous spider naevi can appear suddenly over the upper trunk and face.

Features not described in Bill:

- Gynaecomastia, secondary to testicular atrophy
- Leukonychia (white nails) – also seen in other chronic diseases, e.g. diabetes mellitus
- Finger clubbing, complex mechanism related to venous shunting – more often seen in lung cancer or chronic respiratory disorders
- Asterixis – in advanced liver failure (acute or chronic).

Question 12

What is the likely cause of Bill's haematemesis?

Answer 12

Bleeding oesophageal varices due to portal hypertension. The portal venous pressure of 28 mmHg is not high enough to propel blood through liver sinusoids distorted by fibrous scars.

Sites at which portal–systemic links occur in order to bypass a cirrhotic liver are:

- Lower oesophagus (left gastric and azygos veins). Oesophageal varices rupture easily. Mortality is 50 per cent for each bleeding episode.
- Peri-umbilical region 'caput medusae' (falciform ligament and abdominal veins)
- Retroperitoneum (mesenteric and retroperitoneal veins)
- Superior and inferior rectal veins (haemorrhoids).

The liver biopsy result is that of primary hepatocellular carcinoma arising in a cirrhotic liver.

At Bill's funeral five months later, Malcolm considers how easily he could have shared Bill's fate.

Question 13

When does hepatocellular carcinoma (HCC) usually arise?

Answer 13

There is usually cirrhosis. Risk of HCC is highest in hepatitis B (especially if HBeAg+), alcohol (10–15 per cent of alcoholic cirrhosis) and haemochromatosis. HCC is generally fatal within a year of diagnosis.

Question 14

Why else might a patient with advanced cirrhosis die due to his liver disease?

Answer 14

- Hypovolaemic shock from bleeding varices
- Hepatic encephalopathy, often due to sustained oozing of blood into gastrointestinal tract secondary to coagulopathy
- Spontaneous bacterial peritonitis
- Systemic infection.

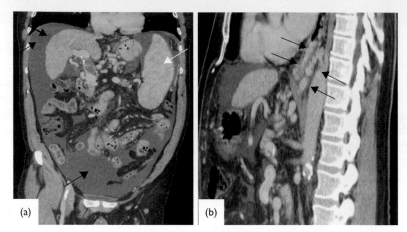

Figure 19.3 (a) Coronal CT in a patient with alcoholic liver disease showing shrunken liver (arrowhead), splenomegaly (white arrow) from portal venous hypertension, and ascites (black arrows). (b) Sagittal view: Note the oesophageal varices (arrows).

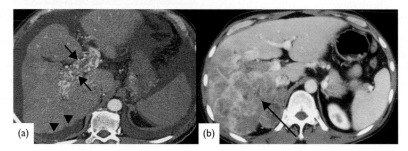

Figure 19.4 (a) CT scan showing hepatocellular carcinoma in a patient with alcoholic liver disease with hypervascular tumour thrombus occluding the portal vein (arrows). Note the nodular margin of the cirrhotic liver (arrowheads) (b) T_1-weighted gradient echo MR post-gadolinium showing an infiltrating hepatocellular carcinoma (arrow) of the right lobe of liver.

Maureen Fitzwilliam, a stoical 73-year-old woman, complains to her GP of gnawing epigastric pain. Previously, her only problems have been osteoarthritis of the knees and hips, for which she takes ibuprofen. She has had 'indigestion' for some weeks. The pain began four days ago. It never eases, even at night. Eating exacerbates it, especially spicy food. Fats such as yoghurt and milk help slightly. On examination, her mucous membranes are slightly pale. The GP suggests that she might have acid reflux into her oesophagus, or possibly gastritis, and prescribes a proton pump inhibitor (PPI).

A day later, she re-presents with nausea, having vomited twice. On questioning she says that the vomit contained dark granular material, like coffee grounds. The GP refers her for urgent endoscopic examination of her oesophagus, stomach and duodenum, which is performed that day on the 'emergency upper GI bleeds' list in the local hospital. A 2-cm-diameter gastric ulcer is noted at the incisura, on the lesser curve. The ulcer edges overhang a rather smooth and clean-looking base, from which a blood vessel protrudes. The endoscopist seals it using diathermy and glue. Several biopsies are taken from the ulcer edge.

Maureen asks why she has developed an ulcer. The doctor explains that anything which damages the stomach's protective coating can allow acid or enzymes to attack it. For instance, she has been taking ibuprofen, a non-steroidal anti-inflammatory drug (NSAID), which can damage the stomach lining. Maureen protests that she has taken ibuprofen for years without harm. The doctor tells her that he has performed a urease test on one biopsy to look for *Helicobacter pylori*, another possible cause, and the other biopsies have been sent to pathology for microscopical examination to check there is no malignancy.

Question 1

How does the stomach protect itself from autodigestion by pepsin and acid?

Answer 1

Mucin-secreting gastric epithelial cells secrete a blanket of mucus which coats the sides of the gastric pits and accumulates thickly on the gastric surface, protecting it.

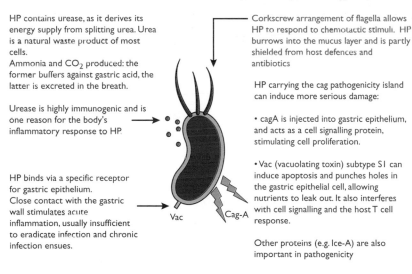

HP contains urease, as it derives its energy supply from splitting urea. Urea is a natural waste product of most cells.
Ammonia and CO_2 produced: the former buffers against gastric acid, the latter is excreted in the breath.

Urease is highly immunogenic and is one reason for the body's inflammatory response to HP.

HP binds via a specific receptor for gastric epithelium.
Close contact with the gastric wall stimulates acute inflammation, usually insufficient to eradicate infection and chronic infection ensues.

Corkscrew arrangement of flagella allows HP to respond to chemotactic stimuli. HP burrows into the mucus layer and is partly shielded from host defences and antibiotics

HP carrying the cag pathogenicity island can induce more serious damage:

• cagA is injected into gastric epithelium, and acts as a cell signalling protein, stimulating cell proliferation.

• Vac (vacuolating toxin) subtype S1 can induce apoptosis and punches holes in the gastric epithelial cell, allowing nutrients to leak out. It also interferes with cell signalling and the host T cell response.

Other proteins (e.g. Ice-A) are also important in pathogenicity

Vac   Cag-A

Clinical points
• The HP breath test is useful for non-invasive HP detection: radiolabelled carbon given orally is detected in the breath if HP are present.
• Antibiotic treatment is effective, but HP can develop resistance quickly so multiple simultaneous therapy is used.
• Vaccines against urease and flagellar antigens are being developed

Figure 20.1 The major features of *Helicobacter pylori* (HP) conferring a survival advantage.

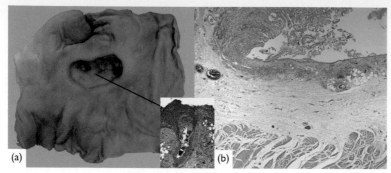

Figure 20.2 (a) Gross features of a peptic ulcer: overhanging, well-demarcated edges and a clean, acid-etched base. This ulcer shows a medium-sized blood vessel at its base (see inset for high-power view). (b) Low-power photomicrograph showing the typical features of a peptic ulcer base lined by acutely inflamed ulcer slough (polymorphs, histiocytes and fibrin) beneath which is granulation tissue. Granulation tissue consists of fibroblasts and new capillaries.

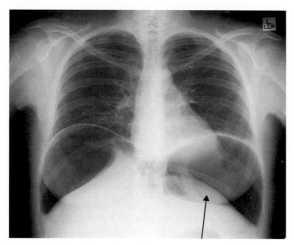

Figure 20.3 Chest X-ray shows free gas (arrow) under the diaphragmatic outlines. This is a sign of a perforated viscus, usually a duodenal ulcer or a diverticulum of the large bowel.

A buffer zone of (alkaline) bicarbonate accumulates between the mucous blanket and the epithelial cells. This is secreted by gastric epithelial cells, stimulated by prostaglandins generated by arachidonic acid breakdown via the cyclo-oxygenase (COX) enzyme pathway (see Figure 2.4).

Pepsinogen is produced by chief cells at the base of the gastric pits in the gastric body and fundus. Hydrochloric acid (HCl) is secreted by cells closer to the neck of the gland than those producing pepsinogen. Pepsinogen is not activated to the active proteolytic enzyme pepsin until it encounters the very low pH acid environment in the gastric lumen.

Question 2

Why are patients taking NSAIDs at risk of peptic ulceration?

Answer 2

NSAIDs block the action of cyclo-oxygenases (they are COX inhibitors) so their use impairs the production of the bicarbonate buffer and increases the risk of acid-induced damage, especially if mucin production is impaired or the mucus layer is breached by food. Patients on long-term NSAIDs are usually also prescribed a PPI to diminish gastric acid production.

Within half an hour the urease test is positive, indicating that the gastric biopsy placed in indicator solution contained *Helicobacter pylori*.

Antibiotics are added to the PPI prescribed by the GP.

Question 3

What is *Helicobacter pylori* and how does it cause disease in the stomach and duodenum?

Answer 3

Helicobacter pylori (HP) is a Gram-negative, curved, flagellate bacterium. It survives the harsh acid environment of the stomach by secreting urease, a urea-splitting enzyme, to surround itself with ammonia. Urea is a waste product of all cells including gastric epithelium.

HP use flagella to burrow through the mucous barrier. They bind to gastric epithelium. Some strains of HP punch holes to obtain nutrients from the gastric cell. This causes acute inflammation, which not only releases

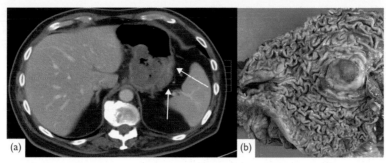

Figure 20.4 (a) CT scan demonstrates thickening of the stomach wall by carcinoma (arrow) in a lesion which resembled a chronic gastric ulcer on endoscopy. (b) An ulcerated gastric cancer which has similarities with a benign peptic ulcer. Biopsy is advised at the edges of any gatric ulcer. Duodenal ulcers are rarely malignant.

further nutrients for the bacteria but also generates further inflammation, which erodes the gastric lining. Damaged gastric epithelium secretes little or no mucin and the mucous layer becomes thinned in these areas. Thus the mucosa is vulnerable to acid and proteolytic degradation.

HCl concentration is lowest in the antrum, because it is made by the body and fundus of the stomach. Its release is stimulated by histamine and gastrin, released by G-cells in the antrum, and is inhibited by somatostatin, released by antral D-cells. HP destroys D-cells and thus removes acid inhibition. Increased gastric HCl production can damage the duodenum (usually the combination of bile and pancreatic enzymes returns the duodenal pH to a normal or mildly alkaline pH). This may cause ulceration.

Depending on the strain of HP encountered and the extent of gastric colonization and damage, the outcome can be very different. Antral HP with high acid output causes >90 per cent of duodenal peptic ulcers, whereas 60–70 per cent of gastric peptic ulcers are due to global colonization of the stomach by HP with widespread gastric atrophy and therefore diminished acid production. However, there must be some acid present or peptic ulcers do not form.

HP is a 'class I carcinogen', i.e. it is strongly implicated in the causation of cancer.

Aggressive strains (e.g. those carrying Vac-A which are able to punch holes in gastric epithelial cells, and those with Cag-A which promote epithelial cell proliferation) may cause severe chronic gastritis. Subsequent intestinal metaplasia predisposes to the development of gastric adenocarcinoma.

Another HP-linked malignancy is MALT-type lymphoma of stomach, which is linked with persistent lymphoid stimulation and certain characteristic mutations.

People with HP either seem to have peptic ulcer-forming strains or cancer-causing strains, thus cancer is rarely a complication of peptic ulcer.

Question 4

What is chronic inflammation and why does it occur in association with HP infection?

Answer 4

Chronic inflammation often occurs when the initiating stimulus cannot be cleared by the acute inflammatory response. It is characterized by lymphocytes, plasma cells and macrophages in the inflammatory infiltrate. Acute (i.e. polymorph-rich) inflammation may also persist, but polymorphs usually disappear as chronic inflammation takes over.

HP is not cleared by the transient acute inflammatory response which it engenders because it activates inflammation remotely, by injuring epithelial cells. After a short acute response, chronic inflammation supervenes and antibodies to HP can be detected in the blood. These persist for some years after the organism has been cleared, so in order to detect active infection a urease test is performed. This detects the action of urease and can be done as a breath test or on a biopsy.

In the breath test, HP urease releases carbon dioxide into the breath when carbon radiolabelled urea is ingested. In the biopsy urease test, a gastric biopsy is placed in an indicator solution, which changes colour as ammonia is produced and the pH increases. A new antibody test for HP can be applied to faecal samples – a quick, easy and cheap test which will probably take the place of breath testing and biopsy.

Question 5

Maureen had clinically obvious bleeding from a large blood vessel at the base of the ulcer. How does upper gastrointestinal tract bleeding present clinically?

Answer 5

Nausea and vomiting of altered blood is typical of a bleeding gastric ulcer. The partly acid-digested blood looks like coffee grounds.

Large amounts of blood may be passed per rectum from either gastric or duodenal ulcers, but by this time the blood has been partly digested and mixed with faeces, producing tarry stools with a distinctive metallic smell, 'melaena'.

If the amount of blood lost per day is slight, it may not be noticed by the patient until symptoms of iron-deficiency anaemia develop (e.g. tiredness, shortness of breath, pale mucous membranes).

Question 6

Why don't all peptic ulcers bleed catastrophically?

Answer 6

Gradual erosion of the wall of the stomach or duodenum with associated chronic inflammation allows time for vessels to close off through a process called 'endarteritis obliterans', a mixture of endothelial and intimal proliferation with thrombosis and fibrosis, which either seals the vessels or reduces bleeding to a minimum.

Question 7

How else may peptic ulcer present clinically?

Answer 7

Retrosternal pain due to erosion of the pancreas, which is retroperitoneal and lies directly behind the stomach.

'Acute abdomen' with severe pain and peritonism due to perforation of the free wall of the duodenum or stomach, with leakage of contents into the peritoneal cavity and chemical peritonitis. A plain abdominal X-ray shows air under the diaphragm.

Maureen asks if she will have to have an operation. When her husband had a duodenal ulcer many years ago he had part of his stomach and duodenum removed. He was never the same again. She is delighted to learn that the ulcer will almost certainly heal by itself, now that she is on the right medication.

Question 8

What type of healing takes place in peptic ulcers?

Answer 8

Peptic ulcers are broad-based, deep, steep-sided holes with overhanging tops, like the edges of cliffs. Figure 20.2a shows a typical example.

Healing is by secondary intention, in which the wound base heals by forming granulation tissue, in which fibrous scar tissue develops – this is 'organization'. The surface epithelium proliferates and regenerates over the top, but a broad scar links the smooth muscle and submucosal edges. The scar tissue contracts, reducing the size of the wound (see Figure 42.4). (Healing by primary intention (see Figure 42.3) occurs if the wound edges can be brought together, for instance the incisional wound made at surgical operation, which produces less scarring.)

Question 9

What can interfere with the healing of ulcers?

Answer 9

- Persistence of the initial stimulus (so it is important to stop NSAIDs or treat HP).
- Deficiency of vitamin C or zinc, important for collagen formation.

CASE 21

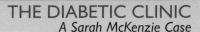

One of the first outpatient clinics that Sarah McKenzie had attended when she had started the clinical part of her undergraduate training was a diabetic clinic. A visit to the diabetic clinic was part of the introductory fortnight that took place before the students were allocated to the rotation between the various specialties that formed the bulk of the first clinical year. Armed only with knowledge of normal endocrine physiology, she had found the experience quite daunting.

A month on and now attached to the endocrinology team, her current concept of diabetes was one of a swirling myriad of different forms and doses of insulin darting about like ethereal shadows existing only as tantalizing forms on the edges of her perception where they danced with the taunting imp that was HbA1c and the jagged acronymic ghouls of DKA and HONKDC.

The endocrinology specialist registrar broke Sarah out of her nightmarish contemplation and jolted her back into firm reality.

'Hi, I'm Jim Plant, you're nice and early. That'll give us a few minutes to set the scene before the patients start coming in.'

'Definitions of a disease are a good place to start,' said Dr Plant. 'If you have a good definition, that'll often tell you a lot about the disease. So, how would you define diabetes?'

Sarah had been preparing hard for this firm and had also received some lectures about diabetes from the pathology department, so she was ready for this question. 'Diabetes is a condition in which there is either a deficiency in the production of, or a decreased sensitivity to insulin.'

'Yep, that about encapsulates it. Are there any subtypes?'

'Type 1 and type 2,' Sarah forged ahead confidently.

'And how are they different?'

'In type 1 the body fails to make insulin. In type 2, there is insulin secretion, but it's either at a decreased level or there's resistance to its effects.'

'That's good. How else are they known?'

'Type 1 is insulin dependent, because patients have to be given exogenous insulin. Type 2 is non-insulin dependent, because it can usually be managed without exogenous insulin.'

'Excellent. Don't forget secondary causes of diabetes either. If need be, you can work those out from basic glucose physiology. Any offers?'

Sarah already had a list in her head, but was grateful for the memory aid. 'Cushing's syndrome, exogenous corticosteroids, acromegaly, thyrotoxicosis, phaeochromocytoma, pancreatic surgery, chronic pancreatitis and tropical diabetes.'

'That's pretty comprehensive. In chronic pancreatitis, the islets of Langerhans are often quite resistant relative to all the chaos that's going on around them, but they're not invulnerable. Just a couple more things before we see the next patient. What's the main fundamental consequence of diabetes mellitus?'

'Raised blood glucose,' answered Sarah.

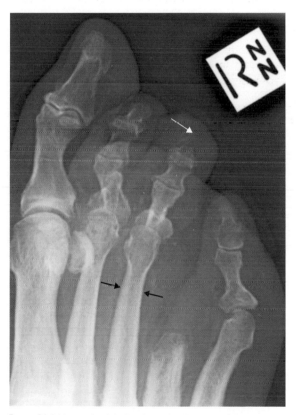

Figure 21.1 X-ray of a right forefoot in a diabetic patient showing vascular calcification of the small vessels of the foot, indicating atherosclerosis (arrow). The fourth toe has been amputated because of a previous episode of gangrene. There is destruction of the distal phalanx of the third toe (white arrow) because of osteomyelitis complicating an ulcerated toe – a result of the loss of sensation accompanying diabetic neuropathy and impaired healing because of a poor blood supply.

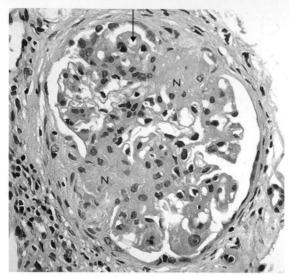

Figure 21.2 High-power photomicrograph from a kidney with diabetic glomerulopathy showing the 'Kimmelstein Wilson' kidney, with thickening of the basement membrane (arrow) and nodular thickening of the mesangial cells (N), the cells which support the glomerular tuft.

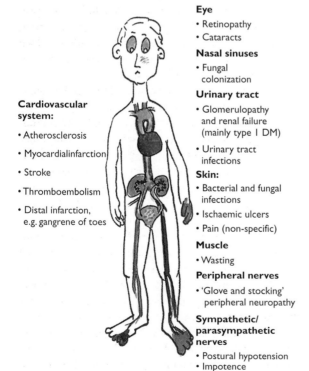

Eye
- Retinopathy
- Cataracts

Nasal sinuses
- Fungal colonization

Urinary tract
- Glomerulopathy and renal failure (mainly type I DM)
- Urinary tract infections

Skin:
- Bacterial and fungal infections
- Ischaemic ulcers
- Pain (non-specific)

Muscle
- Wasting

Peripheral nerves
- 'Glove and stocking' peripheral neuropathy

Sympathetic/ parasympathetic nerves
- Postural hypotension
- Impotence

Cardiovascular system:
- Atherosclerosis
- Myocardialinfarction
- Stroke
- Thromboembolism
- Distal infarction, e.g. gangrene of toes

Figure 21.3 Summary of the many clinical problems associated with diabetes mellitus. Their onset may be deferred or prevented by good control of blood glucose levels.

'And there are assorted consequences to that, which we'll probably see in the clinic, unfortunately for the patients. What other metabolic pathways are affected?'

Sarah was still in territory that was familiar to her. 'Insulin is a metabolic hormone that helps the body to deal with nutritional loads after meals. It increases the uptake of glucose, amino acids and fatty acids into cells and promotes their storage by increasing the synthesis of glycogen, proteins, triglycerides and cholesterol and generally inhibiting their breakdown.'

'That's a good starting point. You can also think of it as an anabolic hormone. Okay, last thing before we start. We won't be seeing anybody with a diabetic ketoacidosis or hyperosmolar, non-ketotic coma today, but do you know why type 1 diabetics get DKAs [diabetic ketoacidosis] and type 2s have HONKs [hyperosmolar non-ketotic coma]?'

Sarah knew this was the case but had never established why.

'It's in the answer you just gave,' explained Dr Plant. 'Insulin inhibits the production of ketones. People with type 1 diabetes don't have any, so ketone production is unchecked. Type 2 patients still have enough to suppress ketone bodies. Right, that's enough of the theory, let's see our first patient. He's one of our regulars, 62 years old, very nice chap, his control isn't too bad but it could be better and unfortunately he used to smoke for 20 years after diagnosis. He stopped two years ago. Now, write down on this piece of paper what complication of his diabetes you think he's most likely to have suffered. We'll call him in once you've done that and see if you're right afterwards.'

Dr Plant invited the patient into the clinic. The consultation was fairly quick as the patient required only a basic follow-up. 'Before you go, can I just ask you to tell Sarah what happened to you in April two years ago, please?' Dr Plant requested the patient.

'Sure. I had a heart attack. Well, myocardial infarction, that was the medical term I think. Luckily I got to hospital quickly and it wasn't as bad as it could have been, but it gave me a wake-up call and I stopped smoking.'

Dr Plant thanked the patient and wished him goodbye.

'So, what did you go for?' wondered Dr Plant with a grin as he opened the paper. 'Atherosclerosis. Well done. Why did you say that?'

'Diabetes is a risk factor for atherosclerosis and so is smoking. The combination of the two is very bad.'

'Absolutely. Why does diabetes cause atherosclerosis?'

'You can get hyperlipidaemia but it's thought that the raised blood glucose and abnormal glycosylation of proteins damages the endothelium directly.'

'Yes. That's a useful phrase, "abnormal glycosylation of proteins". At present, it gets you out of a lot of awkward pathogenic questions in diabetes. Do you know any practical use of it?'

Sarah had not been relishing this question as it involved one of her foes, HbA1c. 'It's something to do with HbA1c, but I'm not sure how.'

Dr Plant smiled, as if he was recalling his own time as a student. 'That's the key word. HbA1c is a glycosylated form of haemoglobin. The higher your average blood glucose is over time, the greater the percentage of haemoglobin that is in this glycosylated form. Non-diabetics have some but people with diabetes are at risk of having abnormally high levels, unless their glucose levels are well controlled. Because HbA1c levels reflect the overall glucose level over the previous few weeks, it's a good test for measuring the overall control over this period. A one-off pinprick or other blood test only tells you about the glucose there and then. The long-term control is what's important for the long-term complications.'

'I think I understand,' said Sarah, pondering the information.

'Reviewing the HbA1c and the patient's own finger prick glucose levels chart is one of the key parts of the clinic,' added Dr Plant. 'If they're not as good as they should be, you want to tighten up the control, either by adjusting the dose or its timing or frequency. That's something that comes with practice. It often seems very confusing as a student, but just be aware of the principles of insulin use.'

'Ah, the next patient should have some signs,' observed Dr Plant as he reviewed the next set of notes. 'Why don't you take her into the side room and examine the fundi and also do a neurological examination of her arms and lower limbs. Just concentrate on below the elbows and knees for the motor side of things. While you're doing that I'll see these couple of straightforward follow-ups.'

Sarah went into the side room and one of the clinic assistants brought the patient into her. Sarah spent a few minutes with the patient, then returned to Dr Plant to present her findings.

'Mrs Bartholomew is a 63-year-old woman who's had type 2 diabetes for 20 years. When I looked in her fundi, I couldn't see too much and I'm afraid that I couldn't find anything wrong.'

'That's okay, don't worry. We'll see what we can do about that. What about her limbs?'

'Her tone, power and co-ordination were normal. I could get her upper limb reflexes but not her ankle jerks or plantars. She had impaired sensation for crude touch, fine touch and proprioception in the distal parts of her fingers and over all of her toes and back to the middle of her foot.'

'Was it symmetrical or not?'

Sarah thought for a couple of seconds. 'Symmetrical.'

'Do you know what name's given to that distribution?'

'Glove and stocking.'

'Yes. It's not the only pattern of neuropathy that patients with diabetes get, but it's one of the classic ones. Why do people with diabetes get neuropathy?'

'Abnormal glycosylation of proteins?' hazarded Sarah, although she could not help herself from smiling as she felt at ease with Dr Plant.

Dr Plant laughed. 'See, it's a piece of cake. Of course, I should have discussed sorbitol with you earlier. It's a metabolite of glucose and if there's more glucose around, there'll be more sorbitol. Sorbitol is toxic to a variety of tissues, including nerves and is thought to be very important in the neuropathy. And to be really precise, we need to distinguish between glycosylation, which is enzyme dependent and glycation, which doesn't need enzymes. Now, let's take a look at Mrs Bartholomew's fundi again.'

Dr Plant took Sarah back to see Mrs Bartholomew. 'I'm not surprised you couldn't see anything with this,' he declared, inspecting the decrepit, clunky ophthalmoscope that was attached to the wall. 'It's probably older than both of us combined. Luckily, Mrs Bartholomew was seen by the ophthalmologists last week and they've taken some pictures of her retina. We'll take a look at them after we've seen what we can do for Mrs Bartholomew today.'

Dr Plant and Sarah returned to the main room. Dr Plant opened Mrs Bartholomew's notes and showed Sarah two retinal photographs. 'These are much better than fundoscopy,' explained Dr Plant. 'These are what you see in the textbooks and nobody ever explains to you that fundoscopy gives you a much smaller field of view unless you move the scope around. So you see pictures like these, then do fundoscopy and think that you're rubbish at it, which isn't true. I'll run through the changes for you, just so you can get your eye in. There's a microaneurysm there, a small haemorrhage there, a cotton wool spot there and these two things are hard exudates. These are all non-proliferative changes. Luckily for Mrs Bartholomew, she hasn't got any proliferative retinopathy yet. That's the really serious thing because vitreous haemorrhage, visual loss and retinal detachment can occur.'

'Is that related to the things we've already discussed?'

'Yes. Sorbitol metabolism, glycosylation and glycation. It's also an example of how diabetes causes microvascular disease. Atherosclerosis is more of a larger vessel process, whereas diabetic neuropathy, retinopathy and one other complication you'll tell me in a minute, are classified as microvascular. So, what's that one other?'

'Diabetic nephropathy.'

'Which manifests as what pattern of renal disease ultimately?'

'Nephrotic syndrome,' offered Sarah.

'Why do you say that?'

'Because you start off with microalbuminuria, which gets worse and worse, so at some point the protein loss reaches nephrotic levels.'

'That's it. If we add in cataracts, probably our friend sorbitol again, that's pretty much diabetes in essence, barring the emergencies. So, your key concepts are macro- and microvascular damage/atherosclerosis, the abnormal sticking of glucose molecules onto things, sorbitol being nasty, diabetic neuropathy, retinopathy and nephropathy. Don't forget the increased susceptibility to infection. Add in raised blood glucose, loss of the anabolic effects on protein and fat metabolism, the role of HbA1c in providing an overview of the patient's diabetic control and the importance of good diabetic control in preventing complications and you're pretty much done. The nuances of management come with practice and knowing the basic theory and the tools in the treatment arsenal.'

PART 3

INVESTIGATIONS

A 69-year-old man decides to avail himself of the well-man check-up that his local GP offers for people over the age of 60. He feels that he is in good health and wants to keep things that way. The GP does not find anything untoward on history or examination, but also requests some blood tests and arranges to see the patient in a fortnight to discuss the results. The blood tests are normal, with the exception of the full blood count.

Investigations

Full blood count

Hb	11.4 g/dL
WCC	6.2×10^9/L
Platelets	291×10^9/L
MCV	103 fL
MHC	32.4 pg
MCHC	34.0 g/dL

Question 1

What abnormality is present?

Answer 1

The patient has macrocytic anaemia.

Question 2

What are the causes of macrocytosis?

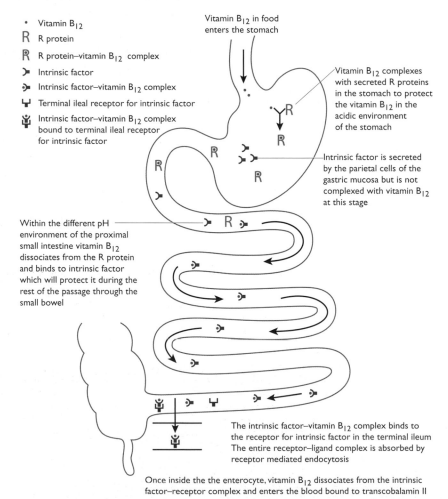

Figure 22.1 Mechanism of absorption of vitamin B_{12}.

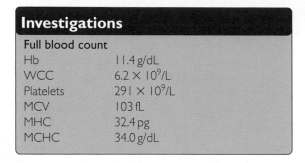

- •   Vitamin B_{12}
- R   R protein
- R   R protein–vitamin B_{12} complex
- ⋗   Intrinsic factor
- ⋗   Intrinsic factor–vitamin B_{12} complex
- ⊔   Terminal ileal receptor for intrinsic factor
- ⋓   Intrinsic factor–vitamin B_{12} complex bound to terminal ileal receptor for intrinsic factor

Vitamin B_{12} in food enters the stomach

Vitamin B_{12} complexes with secreted R proteins in the stomach to protect the vitamin B_{12} in the acidic environment of the stomach

Intrinsic factor is secreted by the parietal cells of the gastric mucosa but is not complexed with vitamin B_{12} at this stage

Within the different pH environment of the proximal small intestine vitamin B_{12} dissociates from the R protein and binds to intrinsic factor which will protect it during the rest of the passage through the small bowel

The intrinsic factor–vitamin B_{12} complex binds to the receptor for intrinsic factor in the terminal ileum The entire receptor–ligand complex is absorbed by receptor mediated endocytosis

Once inside the the enterocyte, vitamin B_{12} dissociates from the intrinsic factor–receptor complex and enters the blood bound to transcobalamin II

Answer 2

- Vitamin B_{12} deficiency
- Folate deficiency
- Alcohol
- Hypothyroidism
- Aplastic anaemia
- Haemolysis
- Myelodysplasia
- Myeloma
- Pregnancy
- Cytosine
- Mercaptopurine.

Question 3

What simple investigation could be carried out next?

Answer 3

The simplest next step that has a good chance of uncovering the cause of the patient's macrocytic anaemia is a blood test for folate and vitamin B_{12} levels.

Question 4

The GP arranges the blood test. The man has normal folate levels, but a reduced vitamin B_{12}. How is vitamin B_{12} absorbed?

Answer 4

The body has a specific system for the absorption of vitamin B_{12}. In order to protect the vitamin B_{12} (cobalamin) molecule in the digestive environment of the gastrointestinal tract, it is first complexed with R proteins in the lumen of the stomach. These remain bound to the vitamin B_{12} until the small intestine, where the different luminal conditions favour the binding of vitamin B_{12} to intrinsic factor (IF). Intrinsic factor is synthesized by the parietal cells of the stomach.

The vitamin B_{12} intrinsic factor complex passes along the small intestine until it reaches the terminal ileum. The enterocytes in the terminal ileum possess special receptors that permit receptor-mediated endocytosis of the vitamin B_{12}–intrinsic factor complex. The complex is then transported across the enterocyte and the vitamin B_{12} is released into the blood now bound to transcobalamin II. Specific receptors for the vitamin B_{12}–transcobalamin II complex exist on cells and again mediate receptor-mediated endocytosis. This process is particularly manifested by the liver.

Question 5

What conditions could cause a deficiency of vitamin B_{12}?

Answer 5

Most conditions in which the body has either reduced or elevated levels of a nutrient can be considered in terms of intake, absorption, metabolism/distribution and excretion. In the case of vitamin B_{12}, the disease states relate mainly to the absorption aspect.

Vitamin B_{12} is found mainly in animal products, so the vegan diet is especially susceptible to being deficient

Table 22.1 Conditions causing vitamin B_{12} deficiency	
Decreased intake	Vegan diet
Impaired absorption	Pernicious anaemia
	Gastrectomy
	Bacterial overgrowth
	Tropical sprue
	Fish tapeworm
	Coeliac disease (rare as a cause of vitamin B_{12} deficiency)
	Crohn's disease
	Ileal disease/resection
	Chronic pancreatic disease
	Zollinger–Ellison syndrome (rare)
	Transcobalamin disorders (rare)
Increased metabolism	Pregnancy
	Haemolysis
	Disseminated malignancy

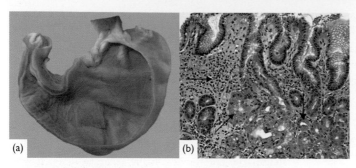

Figure 22.2 Atrophy of the gastric glands. (a) The mucosal lining lacks the usual rugal folds of a normal stomach and is featureless. (b) Microscopy of gastric body mucosa shows chronic inflammation and atrophy of specialized glands in some areas (black arrow). Some residual gastric pits contain specialized parietal cells (red arrow), which secrete acid and intrinsic factor, and chief cells (blue arrow), which secrete pepsinogen.

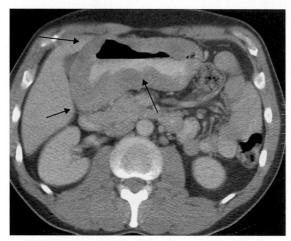

Figure 22.3 CT shows a diffusely infiltrating gastric carcinoma of the body and antrum of the stomach (arrows). Pernicious anaemia can result in polyps and dysplastic change in the gastric epithelium and is a risk factor in the development of gastric cancer.

in vitamin B_{12}. The gastric parietal cells are the source of IF. If these cells are destroyed or otherwise lost, inadequate levels of IF are available to permit the absorption of vitamin B_{12}. Unlike many other nutrients, the absorption of vitamin B_{12} is restricted to the terminal ileum, rather than occurring throughout the small bowel. Therefore, diseases of the terminal ileum will disrupt the absorption of vitamin B_{12}.

A more comprehensive list is given in Table 22.1.

Question 6

What further investigations could determine the cause of the vitamin B_{12} deficiency?

Answer 6

There are several tests that could be performed, but one method involves giving the patient an oral dose of radiolabelled vitamin B_{12}. Once adequate time for absorption

has been allowed, the quantity of the dose that has been absorbed can be measured. This can be done either with sophisticated nuclear medicine scanning of the body, or by the use of an intramuscular injection of a large dose of unlabelled vitamin B_{12} to flush the radiolabelled vitamin B_{12} into the urine, where it can be quantified. The procedure is then repeated with the addition of intrinsic factor with the oral radiolabelled vitamin B_{12}.

In dietary deficiency, absorption is normal without and with intrinsic factor. In deficiencies of IF, absorption is reduced with vitamin B_{12} alone, but is corrected with the co-administration of IF. If the problem is in the terminal ileum, absorption is defective both times.

Question 7

The patient undergoes some further investigations and is found to have reduced absorption of vitamin B_{12} that is corrected by the administration of IF. Given that he has not had a gastrectomy, what is the diagnosis and what is its pathogenesis?

Answer 7

The patient has pernicious anaemia. This is an autoimmune condition in which there is a reaction that is directed against the gastric parietal cells of the stomach. Patients have antibodies that are directed against the parietal cells themselves, or IF, or both. Note that a previous gastrectomy would have yielded the same result in the test.

Question 8

What histopathological changes would be expected in the stomach?

Answer 8

The stomach displays a chronic inflammatory cell infiltrate that will feature lymphocytes and plasma cells.

There is atrophy of the gastric glands, due to the destruction of their cells by the autoimmune response. The changes will be most marked in the body of the stomach where the parietal cells are concentrated.

An infiltrate of chronic inflammatory cells in the affected organ(s) is a common feature of autoimmune diseases.

Question 9

As well as the reduction in the output of IF by the stomach, the secretion of what else is decreased in pernicious anaemia?

Answer 9

Gastric acid.

Question 10

How does vitamin B_{12} deficiency cause anaemia?

Answer 10

One of the roles of vitamin B_{12} is the conversion of ribonucleotides into deoxyribonucleotides. It is therefore vital in DNA synthesis. The incredibly high rate of cell turnover in the bone marrow makes it susceptible to a deficiency of vitamin B_{12}. DNA synthesis becomes impaired and this disrupts the maturation of erythrocytes, culminating in the generation of macrocytes (megaloblastic anaemia). Morphological changes are also seen in neutrophils and their precursors. Folate deficiency produces the same features.

Question 11

What other organ system is affected by vitamin B_{12} deficiency?

Answer 11

The central nervous system. Vitamin B_{12} deficiency can cause subacute combined degeneration of the spinal cord in which there is damage to myelin. The precise mechanism is uncertain, but it may relate to the role of vitamin B_{12} in the conversion of methylmalonyl CoA into succinyl CoA. If this process is compromised, fatty acid metabolism is altered and this can affect the myelin, which is a fat-rich substance.

Table 22.2 Clinical consequences of fat- and water-soluble vitamin deficiency

Vitamin	Clinical feature
A (retinol)	Xerophthalmia, night blindness, keratomalacia, follicular keratosis
D (cholecalciferol)	Rickets, osteomalacia
E (α-tocopherol)	Ataxia
K	Bleeding disorders
B_1 (thiamine)	Beriberi
B_2 (riboflavin)	Angular stomatitis
Niacin	Pellagra
B_6 (pyridoxine)	Peripheral neuropathy
Pantothenic acid	
Biotin	Dermatitis
B_{12} (cobalamin)	Megaloblastic anaemia, neurological disorders
Folic acid	Megaloblastic anaemia
C (ascorbic acid)	Scurvy

Adapted from Lydyard et al. (2000) Pathology Integrated: An A–Z of Disease and its Pathogenesis. London: Arnold.

The clinical consequences of other fat- and water-soluble vitamin deficiencies are listed in Table 22.2.

Question 12

What is the treatment for vitamin B_{12} deficiency?

Answer 12

If dietary intake is inadequate, this should be corrected. Any underlying disease, such as a tapeworm, should be treated if possible, but if correction of the defective absorption cannot be accomplished, regular injections of vitamin B_{12} are effective.

Question 13

Which other diseases of the stomach are associated with pernicious anaemia (Figure 22.3)?

Answer 13

There is an increased incidence of gastric adenocarcinoma. Some patients develop multiple superficial polypoid neuroendocrine ('carcinoid') tumours.

A 69-year-old man presents to his GP with a six-month history of lower back pain and increasing lethargy. There are no focal findings on examination. The GP orders a variety of blood tests.

Investigations

Hb	9.2 g/dL
WCC	5.1×10^9/L
Platelets	167×10^9/L
MCV	88 fL
MHC	29.4 pg
MCHC	32.3 g/dL
ESR	120 mm/h
Na$^+$	139 mmol/L
K$^+$	4.9 mmol/L
Urea	8.4 mmol/L
Creatinine	153 µmol/L
Ca^{2+} (corrected)	2.9 mmol/L
ALP	78 IU/L
TSH	2.6 mU/L
T$_4$	110 nmol/L

Question 1

What abnormalities are present?

Answer 1

- Normochromic, normocytic anaemia
- Chronic renal failure
- Hypercalcaemia.

Question 2

What are the causes of hypercalcaemia?

Answer 2

- Hyperparathyroidism
- Malignancy – parathyroid hormone-related protein production by the tumour
- Bone metastases
- Myeloma
- Sarcoidosis
- Other granulomatous conditions
- Exogenous vitamin D
- Thyrotoxicosis
- Addison's disease

- Thiazides
- Lithium
- Milk alkali syndrome
- Familial hypocalcuric hypercalcaemia
- Vitamin A toxicity.

Question 3

The GP suspects a particular diagnosis and orders serum electrophoresis with immunoglobulin levels.

Investigations

IgG	39	(6–13 g/L)
IgA	0.7	(0.8–3 g/L)
IgM	0.3	(0.4–2.5 g/L)

A narrow band IgG paraprotein is present. What is the significance of this?

Answer 3

Electrophoresis separates proteins on the basis of their mass. This is usually depicted graphically as a series of peaks plotted against molecular mass. The size of the peak denotes the quantity of the protein present that has that particular relative moleular mass (RMM).

Each of the five classes of immunoglobulin has a different basic RMM from the other four. However, the circulating immunoglobulins within any class are composed of numerous antibodies that have different target antigens. The specificity of an immunoglobulin for its target is dependent upon the amino acid sequences of its variable regions. The differences in amino acid sequence between antibodies means that under normal circumstances, any given immunoglobulin subtype will be found to have a range of RMMs on electrophoresis, although the size of this range will be narrow relative to the overall basic RMM for that antibody class. Thus the corresponding peak on the electrophoresis graph is not a single, very narrow line, but is somewhat broader.

In the case of this patient, this broadening of the peak for the IgG component is lost and instead there is actually only a narrow band. This implies that the IgG element consists of (or is dominated by) only one particular antibody with one particular RMM. Given that all plasma cells that are derived from the same B cell synthesize the same immunoglobulin and that plasma cells derived from different B cells do not secrete the same immunoglobulins, the finding of a single dominant immunoglobulin indicates that there has been a clonal expansion of a single plasma cell. Hence, the band on the electrophoresis is also referred to as a monoclonal band.

Question 4

What is the likely diagnosis?

Answer 4

Myeloma.

Question 5

What is myeloma and how does its nature relate to the electrophoresis findings?

Answer 5

Myeloma is a malignant, monoclonal proliferation of plasma cells that infiltrate the bone marrow and produce lesions within the bone and/or soft tissue. The lesions within bone are typically lytic.

All the malignant plasma cells in a myeloma are derived from a single ancestor and therefore they all synthesize the same immunoglobulin. As the myeloma grows, the quantity of cells in the myelomatous population becomes sufficient to produce a detectable monoclonal immunoglobulin; hence the paraprotein band. Note that some myelomas make light chains only. Rarely, myelomas do not secrete their immunoglobulins at all.

Question 6

Is the diagnosis definitive on the basis of the above information?

Answer 6

No. While the history and investigations are extremely suggestive of myeloma, formal diagnosis of myeloma requires particular criteria to be met (Table 23.1).

Question 7

What other investigations are required to make the diagnosis?

Answer 7

- Bone marrow aspirate and trephine
- Skeletal survey
- Urine electrophoresis for Bence–Jones proteins.

Table 23.1 Diagnostic criteria table

Major	Plasmacytoma demonstrated by biopsy (plasmacytoma is a tumour of plasma cells) Bone marrow plasmacytosis >30% (plasma cells accounting for over 30% of the cells in the bone marrow) Monoclonal immunoglobulin peak of at least a certain minimum value (IgG >35 g/L, IgA >20 g/L) OR at least 1 g/24 hours of kappa or lambda light chains in the urine
Minor	Bone marrow plasmacytosis of 10–30% Monoclonal immunoglobulin peak less than the major criteria levels Lytic bone lesions Residual normal IgM <0.5 g/L, IgA<1 g/L or IgG <6 g/L (immunoparesis)

Question 8

Figure 23.1 includes three sections from a bone marrow trephine that could have come from this patient. One has been stained for kappa light chain and the other for lambda. What is shown and what is the significance?

Answer 8

The bone marrow is infiltrated by a population of plasma cells that express kappa light chain but not lambda. Any given plasma cell uses only one type of light chain, either

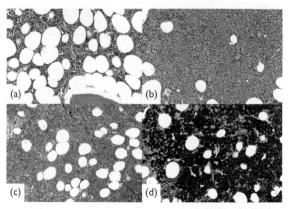

Figure 23.1 (a) Microscopical image of a normal bone marrow (H&E stain). (b) Bone marrow trephine with widespread infiltration by sheets of plasma cells. (c) Immunohistochemistry for lambda light chain in which almost all of the plasma cells are negative. (d) Immunohistochemistry for kappa light chain in which almost all of the plasma cells are positive. The combination of the findings in the kappa and lambda stains indicates that the plasma cells are 'kappa restricted', which implies that they are monoclonal in nature.

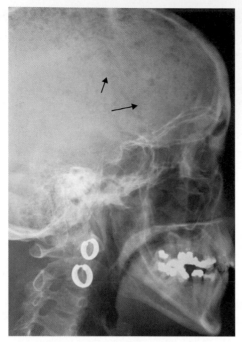

Figure 23.2 Multiple 'punched out' lytic skull vault lesions (arrows) in myeloma.

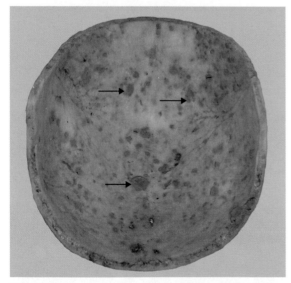

Figure 23.3 Gross photograph showing a skullcap with multiple tumour deposits (arrows), which explain the 'punched out' lytic lesions seen on X-ray.

kappa or lambda, but not both, in the one immunoglobulin it makes. Thus, a normal population of plasma cells should be a mixture of kappa-positive cells and lambda-positive cells. A population which exhibits restriction to one type implies a monoclonal nature.

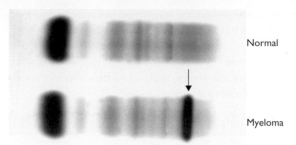

Figure 23.4 Protein electrophoresis shows an 'M-band' (arrowed) in the gamma region of a patient with myeloma, due to secretion of large quantities of a single antibody. A normal patient shows a generalized smear of protein in the gamma region, reflecting the variety of antibodies normally present.

Question 9

What complications can occur in myeloma?

Answer 9

- The lytic deposits of myeloma within bones weaken the structure of the bone and predispose to pathological fractures.
- Osteoclasts are stimulated in myeloma and as well as promoting lysis of bone, their activity releases calcium to the extent that hypercalcaemia develops in 25 per cent of patients who have myeloma.
- Renal failure is encountered in approximately 30 per cent of myeloma patients and has a variety of causes that are sometimes of particular interest to examiners. Light chains are toxic to the renal tubules, where they can precipitate as casts within the tubules. Hypercalcaemia is a cause of renal failure and also increases the risk of renal calculi. Amyloidosis can cause renal failure. If the myeloma causes immuno-compromisation then there may be repeated urinary tract infections and chronic pyelonephritis. The proliferative activity of the myeloma, specifically the nucleic acid metabolism, can elevate serum urate levels, leading to urate nephropathy. The myeloma may infiltrate the kidney (rare). Chemotherapy treatment can be nephrotoxic.
- The excessive production of a clonally derived immunoglobulin can lead to a lack of normal immunoglobulins (immunoparesis). This impairs the immune response.
- The infiltration of the bone marrow by the plasma cells may overwhelm and replace the normal haematopoietic tissue, yielding failure of the bone marrow. The resulting neutropenia can exacerbate the

immunodeficiency. More commonly, the situation is not this severe and only a mild anaemia is found.

- The increased protein content of the blood can cause hyperviscosity. This induces a hypercoaguable tendency, one of the most serious consequences of which is cerebrovascular accident.
- The synthesis of large quantities of immunoglobulin light chains by the myeloma can lead to amyloidosis (AL type).

Question 10

The skull X-ray shown in Figure 23.2 could have come from this patient. What abnormality is present?

Answer 10

The skull features multiple 'punched out' lytic lesions. These are characteristic of myeloma.

SUMMARY

Myeloma is an example of a disease in which the diagnosis requires specific criteria to be met (Table 23.1). In the case of myeloma, all of these criteria are ascertained through specific investigations.

CASE 24

AN ABNORMAL SMEAR TEST

Dr Jones had just been seeing a 40-year-old woman to give her the result of her first cervical smear. The woman was a new patient to the practice and had previously declined invitations to avail herself of the cervical screening programme. The consultation had been a long one because the report for the smear had stated 'suspicious of invasive squamous cell carcinoma' and it had taken some time to deal with matters this raised.

Question 1

Is a report of 'suspicious of invasive squamous cell carcinoma' a typical finding in the cervical screening programme?

Answer 1

Most patients screened will not have a suspicious smear. The purpose of the screening programme is to detect patients who have a precursor lesion that places them at risk of developing cervical carcinoma in the future, but has not reached the stage of an invasive carcinoma at the time of the smear. Detection of the precursor lesion permits preventative treatment to be instituted. It is unusual (and may reflect poor attendance, poor screening or a fast growing lesion) for the smear to be suspicious of invasive cancer.

Question 2

What is the term given to the precursor lesion for cervical squamous cell carcinoma and what is its nature?

Answer 2

The precursor lesion for cervical squamous cell carcinoma is cervical intraepithelial neoplasia (CIN). Intraepithelial neoplasia is a disorder of growth in which the abnormal cells are confined to the epithelium in which they have arisen. At this juncture, the cells neither invade nor metastasize. Within the epithelium, the neoplastic cells possess cytological abnormalities which are similar, to a greater or lesser extent, to those manifested by the carcinoma. The intraepithelial nature of the process limits the scope for architectural changes.

CIN is divided into three grades, CIN 1, CIN 2 and CIN 3. The severity of the cytological changes and the proportion of the epithelium that they occupy increases from CIN 1 to CIN 3.

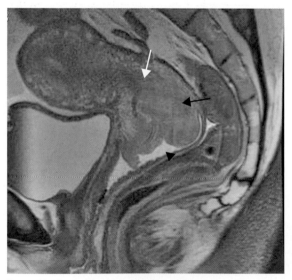

Figure 24.1 Sagittal T$_2$-weighted MRI of a female pelvis showing a cervical squamous cell carcinoma (black arrow) with an exophytic lower margin outlined by fluid/jelly in the vagina (black arrowhead). The tumour obliterates the cervical canal and extends into the lower segment of the uterus (white arrow). The rectum lies posteriorly and the bladder lies anteriorly.

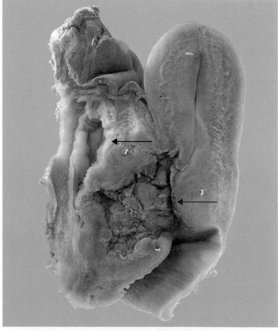

Figure 24.2 Large carcinoma of the anterior part of the cervix (red arrow) which is invading the posterior bladder wall (black arrow).

The thickness cannot be analysed in a smear because the cells are disaggregated. The cells within a smear are assessed for the degree of dyskaryosis that they manifest. Dyskaryosis refers to nuclear cytological abnormalities and does not require the architecture to be evaluated. The grade of dyskaryosis is highly predictive of the grade of CIN and this allows cytology to be the first line of investigation.

The classification and terminology of CIN and dyskaryosis is undergoing revision. In the UK, a three-tier system is retained for both. However, in many other countries a two-tier system of low and high grade has been adopted and CIN has been replaced by squamous intraepithelial lesion.

Question 3

How does the existence of degrees of intraepithelial neoplasia relate to carcinogenesis?

Answer 3

The current model of carcinogenesis proposes that the conversion of a normal cell to a malignant cell which can invade and metastasize requires the accumulation of multiple mutations. As the cell gathers mutations, the alterations to its DNA and behaviour distort its cytological features and pattern and rate of growth more and more, making it and its offspring look increasingly atypical relative to their normal neighbours. Therefore, the classification of intraepithelial neoplasia is an attempt to allocate divisions into this continuum of change where such divisions

provide an indication of how far along the road to malignant transformation the atypical cells have travelled.

In the case of CIN 1, the cells are at an early stage. Progression through to squamous cell carcinoma is low and many cases will regress to normal spontaneously. Conversely, approximately one-third of cases of CIN 3 will evolve into squamous cell carcinoma if action is not taken.

Question 4

What other term is used in some organ systems instead of intraepithelial neoplasia?

Answer 4

The main alternative is dysplasia which prevails in the gastrointestinal tract and in the squamous mucosa of the head and neck organs. Dysplasia literally means a disorder of growth.

Question 5

What options are available in the cervical screening programme if a smear is abnormal?

Answer 5

Cervical smear findings are classified into one of eight categories. The next step in the management is rigidly specified for each of these categories and factors in the results of previous smears. This rigidity is dependent upon the ability of the grade of dyskaryosis to predict the grade of CIN and knowledge of how CIN behaves.

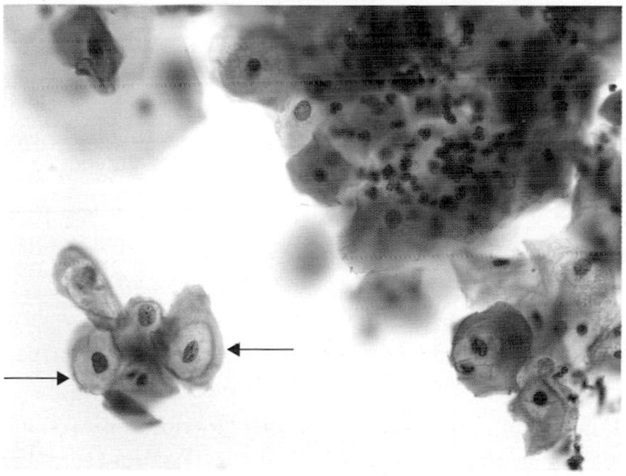

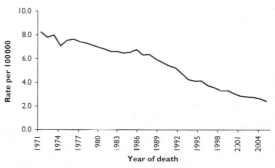

Figure 24.3 Photomicrograph from a smear showing koilocytosis, the typical appearance of cervical squamous cell infected by human papilloma virus (HPV). There is a 'halo' of cleared cytoplasm surrounding an enlarged nucleus (arrow).

Figure 24.4 Age-standardized (European) mortality rates, cervical cancer, UK, 1971–2006. Cervical cancer mortality rates in 2006 (2.4 per 100 000 females) are nearly 70% lower than they were 30 years earlier (7.6 per 100 000 females in 1976). Kindly reproduced from CRC UK (http://info.cancerresearchuk.org/cancerstats/types/cervix/mortality/?a=5441).

For an abnormal smear, the choices are to repeat the smear ahead of the normal recall schedule, to refer to colposcopy, or to refer for a gynaecological opinion.

Colposcopy is the process by which the cervix is visualized under magnification. It views the transformation zone, which is the region of the cervix in which squamous neoplasia tends to arise. In skilled hands, colposcopy can detect a very high proportion of abnormalities and grade them reliably. However, colposcopy does not allow good examination of the endocervical canal, endometrium or ovaries. All of these sites are places in which glandular neoplasms can lurk and shed cells into a smear. Therefore, if a glandular abnormality is detected on a smear, a broader territory must be investigated in order to find the source, necessitating referral for a gynaecological opinion at the outset, rather than just colposcopy.

Question 6

Returning to the patient, given that the GP is referring her for colposcopy, what other investigations are necessary?

Answer 6

The first step is to confirm the suspicion raised by the smear. This will involve a biopsy of the cervix. The biopsy is likely to be in the form of a long loop excision of the transformation zone (LLETZ). A well-taken LLETZ can be 20 mm or more in diameter and for small tumours can remove a large portion of the carcinoma, if not all of it (whether or not the excision is adequate is a separate issue).

Once the diagnosis of squamous cell carcinoma has been confirmed, staging of the tumour is essential. The earliest stages of cervical carcinoma are subdivided to quite a considerable degree and distinction between these substages can be made in a good LLETZ specimen. However, for larger tumours and even for smaller ones that seem to be confined to a LLETZ, imaging studies are necessary to supplement the histological impression.

Imaging is a cornerstone of the staging of most malignant tumours. The choice of imaging that is employed and the regions that must be covered is governed by knowledge of the typical pattern of spread of the tumour. Imaging also has a vital role in planning surgery.

Question 7

To where does cervical carcinoma spread?

Answer 7

The spread of all carcinomas can be considered in the categories of direct extension, local lymph nodes and distant metastases. The direct extension of a cervical carcinoma can be up the endocervical canal and into the body of the uterus, down into the vagina, anteriorly into the bladder or urethra, posteriorly into the rectum and laterally to the pelvic side wall. The ureters can also become invaded by posterolateral extension. The local lymph nodes are the iliac nodes. These will ultimately drain into the para-aortic lymph nodes. Distant metastases in cervical carcinoma are usually to the lungs. Armed with this knowledge, it can be seen that detailed imaging of the pelvis is necessary, supplemented by that of the abdomen and lungs.

Question 8

What is the main risk factor for the development of cervical squamous cell carcinoma?

Answer 8

Infection with high-risk subtypes (including 16, 18, 31 and 33) of the human papilloma virus (HPV). Most of the other risk factors that have been described operate by increasing the chances of acquiring cervical infection with HPV.

Question 9

What is the significance of the patient's smear history in this case?

Answer 9

Entry into the cervical smear programme is around the age of 25, in that this is when women are first issued with invitations to have a smear. This age is chosen as it reflects that at which a significant number of women are developing lesions of CIN but precedes the peak incidence of squamous cell carcinoma. The so-called 'protective effect' of a negative smear is said to be 3–5 years and means that if a woman has a negative cervical smear, she should not develop cervical squamous cell carcinoma in this ensuing time period. In the case of this patient, she had not had any previous smears and therefore there was no opportunity to intercept the carcinoma while it was still at the CIN stage.

Mrs Coleman, a 55-year-old woman had a routine mammogram (Figure 25.1a) as part of the breast cancer screening programme.

Question 1

What does the X-ray show? How does it differ from Figure 25.1b?

Answer 1

Figure 25.1a shows a small cluster of microcalcification. It is suspicious but not sufficiently abnormal to be confident that it represents a malignant lesion. In contrast, Figure 25.1b shows benign calcifications, the thin arrow shows calcification within a blood vessel wall and the thick arrow shows coarse calcification, probably as a result of degenerative changes within the stroma.

Question 2

What will you do next with Mrs Coleman?

Answer 2

Since the calcifications are equivocal and cannot be dismissed as benign, she needs a tissue diagnosis. This can be

done using an fine needle aspiration (FNA) biopsy or by a core needle biopsy (CNB). Since this is a very small area of calcification, it will have to be localized radiologically to make sure the needle goes to the right place.

Mrs Coleman underwent a CNB procedure and the tissue cores were X-rayed (to confirm that there is microcalcification in them) and submitted for histological examination by the pathologist (Figure 25.2).

Question 3

What is the abnormality and hence the diagnosis?

Answer 3

The low-power view of the core biopsy (Figure 25.2a) shows fibro-fatty breast tissue together with ducts showing calcification and expanded by proliferations

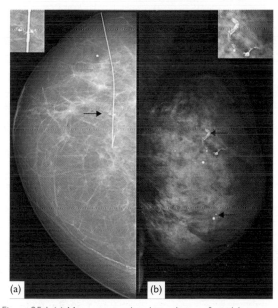

Figure 25.1 (a) Mammogram showing a cluster of suspicious microcalcifications (arrow) which may require a core biopsy to exclude malignancy. In contrast (b) shows benign vascular calcification (red arrow) and benign degenerative coarse stromal calcifications (blue arrow).

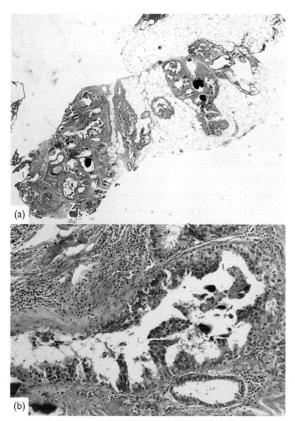

Figure 25.2 (a) Low-power view of core biopsy showing fibro-fatty breast tissue together with ducts showing calcification. (b) Higher power view showing duct expanded by proliferations with micropapillary architecture.

with micropapillary architecture. At higher power (Figure 25.2b), the architecture and the cytological appearances are of a neoplastic proliferation rather than a benign hyperplastic lesion – although it is not entirely straightforward. The cells are confined within the duct and have not broken out of the duct – hence, overall, the features are of a ductal carcinoma in situ (DCIS). The nuclear grade (how much it varies from normal epithelial cells) is low (or well differentiated). Dystrophic calcification occurs within secretions or following degeneration or cell death and hence the pick up on mammography. So, in summary, she has a low-grade DCIS without invasive carcinoma.

Question 4

What other type of in-situ carcinomas do you know?

Answer 4

Lobular carcinoma in situ (LCIS). Despite the similar terminology, the biology of the lesions is quite different. Both types are thought to progress to invasive carcinoma in some women (i.e. they behave as precursor lesions), but unlike DCIS which is usually a unilateral and segmental disease (arising within a localized portion of the breast), LCIS is often multifocal within the breast and occasionally bilateral – hence the risk of invasive carcinoma is also bilateral.

Question 5

The result of Mrs Coleman's biopsy has been transmitted to the surgeon. What will the surgeon do next?

Answer 5

The abnormality needs to be excised. The radiologist will localize the lesion using mammography and place a guidewire near the lesion. This is inserted through the skin and has a small hook on the end to keep it in place. Later the patient will go to theatre and the surgeon will operate and take tissue from around the wire. Following surgery, the specimen will be X-rayed to

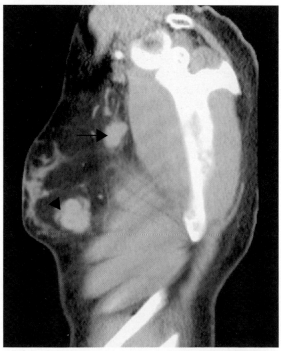

Figure 25.3 Sagittal CT showing a breast mass (arrowhead) with a metastasis in an axillary lymph node (arrow). CT is used currently as a staging tool in breast cancer although positron emission tomography–computed tomography (PET-CT) is taking over this role.

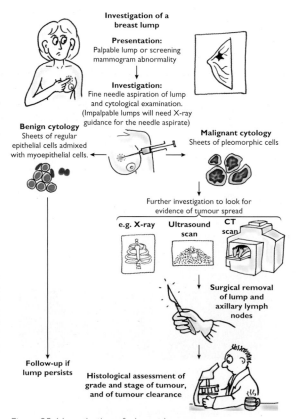

Figure 25.4 Investigation of a breast lump.

make sure the lesion has been excised and the guidewire is in the correct place.

Question 6

The following report was issued by the pathologist after examination of the excisional specimen:

Sections show low-grade ductal carcinoma in situ with microcalcification, measuring 12 mm in maximum dimension. No invasive carcinoma is seen. The lesion extends to medial and inferior margins of the specimen but the rest of the margins are well clear.

What is the most striking information in the report?

Answer 6

The lesion is much bigger than anticipated on the screening mammogram and is still incompletely excised.

Question 7

What does this tell you about the strengths and weaknesses of screening programmes?

Answer 7

Screening programmes are designed to pick up abnormalities before they are clinically symptomatic and hence pick up cancers at an earlier stage. The idea is that this will allow the tumour to be resected while it is still small and with less risk of having metastases and hence, mortality will be reduced. There is little doubt that breast screening programmes have helped to reduce mortality although the exact impact is hotly debated. As with this case, it does cause clinical dilemmas where calcifications of unknown significance are picked up and in a proportion of women, these will be entirely benign, yet the woman will have been subjected to an operative procedure. Further, our ability to predict which precancerous lesion of this type (in-situ carcinomas and atypical hyperplasia) will progress and over what time period is poor. Although she has a diagnosis of a DCIS, it is difficult to predict whether she would have developed an invasive carcinoma and over what time-frame. Current estimates suggest that about 50 per cent will go on to get an invasive cancer but over a 30-year time period. This tumour is at the margins and the size is a surprise. It is clear that not all DCIS or proliferative disease will calcify and it is easy to underestimate the size of lesions. This is also true of invasive carcinoma of lobular type, which grows diffusely and infiltrates as single cells.

Question 8

What will the surgeon do now?

Answer 8

He has to excise further, but since there is nothing to see on radiology and nothing to feel, he has to operate 'blind' by excising all around the previous cavity. If there is further DCIS and it is excised, all is well, but if there is more DCIS and at the margins, he may be forced to do a mastectomy since it is not possible to keep on going back for a little more tissue each time. This is a real scenario that some women with low-grade DCIS are faced with and one of the 'side-effects' of the screening programme — a woman having a mastectomy (a large mutilating operation) for a low-grade, pre-invasive disease!

A 41-year-old mother gives birth to a live male infant at 39 weeks' gestation by spontaneous vaginal delivery. She has had two previous pregnancies, both of which resulted in spontaneous vaginal deliveries of single live neonates at term. Both of these children are healthy and have the same father as the current baby.

Shortly after delivery, the baby seems to be relatively floppy, although he is moving all four limbs and has been crying and responding to stimuli. The baby has also fed successfully. In addition to the hypotonia, examination reveals that the baby's head is particularly round. The palpebral fissures are upward sloping and the medial epicanthal folds are prominent. The tongue is enlarged and heavily fissured. The baby's hands are broad and possess only a single palmar crease, while the little fingers are short and curved inwards. These features persist over the next few months and there is delay in the child reaching the early motor milestones. Later, the child does not learn to walk until the age of three and his speech is delayed until 54 months, although by this time the diagnosis has already been made.

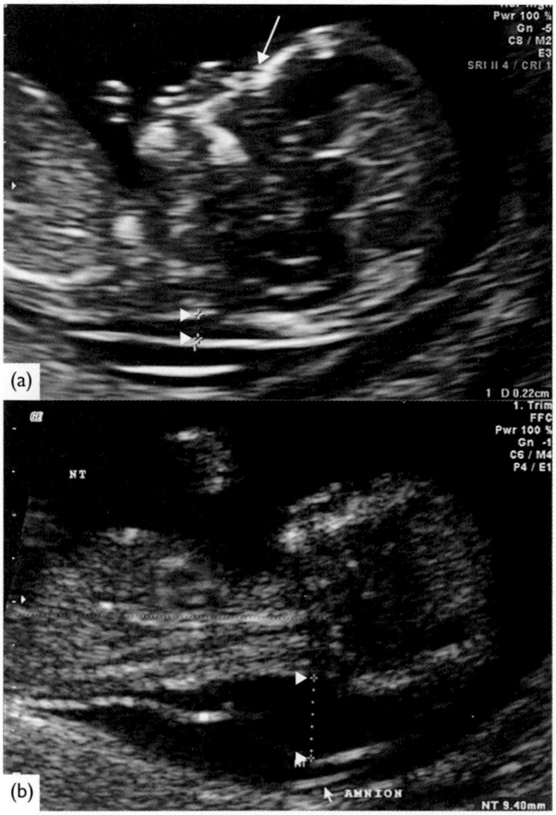

Question 1

What is the diagnosis?

Answer 1

Down syndrome. The physical features are characteristic.

Question 2

What is Down syndrome?

Answer 2

Down syndrome is a chromosomal disorder in which the affected individual has trisomy 21. It should be noted that not all of chromosome 21 needs to be present in excess to produce Down syndrome and that trisomy of a certain portion of the long arm alone will yield the disease.

Figure 26.1 (a) Low-risk and (b) high-risk nuchal translucency (NT) measurement. The NT scan is a screening test which assesses a woman's risk of having a baby with Down syndrome. NT is a normal collection of subcutaneous fluid at the back of a baby's neck. It is measured using ultrasound in terms of thickness (+ … +) at the 11–13 weeks stage of pregnancy.

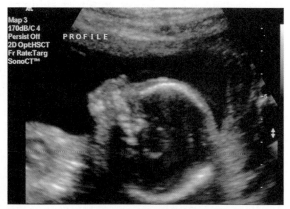

Figure 26.2 Morphology scan performed on a 40-year-old woman. Her 12-week nuchal thickness test gave a 'low risk' of 1 in 500 for Down syndrome. Unfortunately, at this scan there is an abnormal facial profile with a completely absent nasal bone. Significant hypoplasia (<5th percentile) or absent nasal bone may be seen in up to 60% of fetuses with Down syndrome. It is seen in up to 5% of the normal population and variations occur according to race. Note normal nasal bone in Figure 26.1 (white arrow).

Question 3

What is the normal human chromosomal complement?

Answer 3

The normal (euploid) human chromosomal complement is 46. This consists of one pair of sex chromosomes and 22 pairs of autosomes. The normal female has two X chromosomes and the normal male has an X and a Y chromosome.

Question 4

How can an abnormal karyotype arise?

Answer 4

For a person to have an abnormal karyotype requires that either one of the gametes that produced their zygote had an abnormal chromosomal content due to defective meiosis, or that very shortly after division of the zygote there was defective cell mitosis that resulted in duplication of one or more chromosomes that affected all subsequent daughter cells.

Chromosomal diseases normally arise from defective meiosis in the gamete of one or other parent. During meiosis, there is failure of separation of the pair of chromatids. This non-dysjunction means that one of the resulting gametes will have both copies of the chromatids and the other will have neither. Fertilization using these gametes will produce a trisomic or a monosomic disorder respectively.

Question 5

Are chromosomal disorders more likely to have arisen in the mother or father's gametes?

Answer 5

Chromosomal disorders are more common in children born to older mothers. In the case of Down syndrome, the risk becomes particularly significant after the age of 37. This bias towards the maternal gametes reflects the different organization of meiosis in the male and the female. In the male, sperm are generated from their progenitor cells throughout adult life and may therefore be considered to be manufactured fresh. Conversely, females are born with the meiotic production of oocytes already in progress but in a suspended state. These oocytes remain suspended until activated during a menstrual cycle many years later. It is

believed that this renders them more susceptible than sperm to defective meiosis.

Question 6

Other than confirming the diagnosis in the child, is there any other role for postnatal genetic investigation in this family?

Answer 6

Yes. Occasionally (around 3 per cent of cases), Down syndrome results from a balanced (Robertsonian) translocation in one parent. In this situation, the mother has an abnormal karyotype in which the crucial part of one of her chromosome 21s is translocated onto another chromosome. However, she is phenotypically normal because even though the translocated portion of the chromosome is not in the right place, it is still present in each cell in a new location that permits it to function normally. Thus, the cells still retain two copies of all of chromosome 21, just in an abnormal distribution. However, this means that the germ cells also carry the balanced translocation. Therefore, when they undergo meiosis, the shortened chromosome 21 can be separated from the augmented other chromosome that balances it and a gamete results in which a normal chromosome 21 is accompanied by the augmented other chromosome, such that the gamete has a double dose of the long arm of chromosome 21. (Chromosome 14 seems to be susceptible to acquiring the extra part of chromosome 21.)

If a parent has a balanced translocation, they are at particular risk of having another child with Down syndrome because the underlying cause persists. This is in contrast with the majority of cases in which the mutation is sporadic.

Question 7

Given the known increased risk of Down syndrome in older mothers, are there any prenatal screening methods that are available?

Answer 7

A variety of tests can be offered to mothers who are considered to be at risk of having a Down syndrome child.

The fetus synthesizes alpha fetoprotein and some of this enters the maternal blood. In Down syndrome, maternal levels of alpha fetoprotein are low.

Antenatal ultrasound scan performed at 10–14 weeks can measure nuchal thickness (NT). This is a reflection of the amount of fluid in the posterior aspect of the neck and is elevated in Down syndrome. The NT thickness measurement is combined with maternal age and maternal serum assay of PAPP-A (pregnancy-associated plasma protein A) and βhCG (beta human chorionic gonadotrophin). The results are categorized as high risk (>1/300 chance of Down syndrome) or low risk (<1/300 chance). These criteria enable a detection rate of 80–85 per cent with a false-positive rate of 5 per cent.

Neither of these tests is diagnostic and instead they help to estimate the risk that the fetus may have Down syndrome. If the results of the two tests are combined and further integrated with maternal βhCG and oestriol levels, a more accurate prediction of the risk can be obtained, but the result remains a prediction of risk, not a certain diagnosis.

The determination of the specific risk for a given mother is important because the definitive investigation of the possibility of the fetus having Down syndrome requires the invasive procedures of amniocentesis or chorionic villus sampling. In amniocentesis, a volume of amniotic fluid, into which the fetus will have shed cells, is obtained. Chorionic villus sampling involves gathering a sample of placental chorionic villi, which are of fetal origin. The fetal cells can then be cultured and examined in metaphase to display the chromosomes and identify abnormalities of number or structure. In conditions that have a known genetic abnormality, detection of the defective gene in the sampled fetal cells by polymerase chain reaction (PCR) analysis can provide a faster result as it removes the need to culture the cells which is required for a metaphase assessment.

When the diagnosis is made prenatally, the parents may opt for an abortion so it is crucial that the diagnostic test is accurate and specific and this justifies adopting an invasive test. Both amniocentesis and chorionic villus sampling can induce miscarriage. It is therefore important to have as much information available as possible before deciding whether or not this risk is acceptable.

Question 8

What other chromosomal disorders are recognized?

Answer 8

After Down syndrome, the next two most likely chromosomal disorders to be of relevance to undergraduates are Turner syndrome and Klinefelter syndrome. These are both disorders of the sex chromosomes. Turner syndrome patients are all female and have a 45 XO karyotype due to the fact that they lack one X chromosome. Klinefelter syndrome patients are males who are 47 XXY. Beyond these two are Patau syndrome (trisomy 13) and Edwards syndrome (trisomy 18) (which are tested for routinely on amniocentesis samples).

Question 9

What other disease frequently features aneuploidy? Aneuploid cells are those that contain an abnormal number of chromosomes, i.e. not an exact multiple of 23.

Answer 9

Many malignant cells are aneuploid. The gain or loss of particular chromosomes can be an advantage to a cell from the perspective of achieving malignant function. Aneuploidy in carcinogenesis results from defective mitosis.

Sarah McKenzie was not entirely sure what to expect in the genetics outpatient clinic. The consultant, Dr Lucy Barrett, had only been appointed a few weeks earlier and Sarah was one of the very first students to attend the clinic. All Sarah knew was that Dr Barrett was in her early thirties and did not possess an established reputation for making life hard for students. Nevertheless, Sarah remained nervous about the clinic because she always found it hard to remember patterns of inheritance and was not sure what Dr Barrett would be asking her.

Dr Barrett greeted Sarah with a smile when Sarah introduced herself and told her to take a seat.

'A lot of the patients who are coming here today, Sarah, are for genetic counselling of one sort or another. Either they or somebody in their family has a genetic disease and they're understandably concerned about the possibility that their children or another family member might also be at risk. Exactly where we take things from there depends on the disease, its pattern of inheritance and what treatment and screening options there are.'

Sarah nodded in the way that medical students have when they wish to show that they are paying attention without risking having to say anything.

'Take a look at the family tree of this first patient,' said Dr Barrett, passing the patient's notes to Sarah and pointing to a diagram (Figure 27.1a). 'What pattern of inheritance can you see here?'

This was not exactly what Sarah had been expecting, but she was a little relieved because at least she could work the answer out this way. 'It's autosomal dominant,' replied Sarah.

'That's right. What features let you say that?'

'It just looks like it,' said Sarah, a little embarrassed. 'I've never thought about it at a more detailed level.'

Dr Barrett smiled. 'That's okay, a lot of people just look at a family tree and get the right answer without necessarily knowing what steps are going on in their head. In this case, you can see that there are several different generations that are all affected. The disease can be transmitted from either a mother or father to either sons or daughters and every affected person has a parent who has the disease. But you're right, most people, me included, tend to make the decision by pattern recognition, rather than heuristic analysis. Now before we see the patient, do you know what types of disease are autosomal dominant?'

'No,' confessed Sarah, who was quite curious to learn if there was some sort of blanket rule that would make learning modes of inheritance a lot easier.

'Diseases that are due to changes in structural proteins,' informed Dr Barrett. 'It's like building a house. Even if half your bricks are normal, in other words the proteins from the normal allele, if the other 50 per cent of the bricks are defective but are being built into the house all the same, it's going to be an odd house. How odd depends on exactly what the bricks are for.'

The patient was brought into the room and Dr Barrett asked Sarah to go and examine him in a side room while she saw another patient.

Sarah noticed that the patient was very tall and had very long arms. His fingers were long and slender, as were his toes. When Sarah looked in the patient's mouth, his palate was high arched. Examination of the patient's heart revealed a mid-systolic murmur over the apex. Sarah also thought there might have been an early diastolic murmur at the lower left sternal edge, but she was not sure.

'So what do you think's the diagnosis?' inquired Dr Barrett when Sarah reported back.

'Does he have Marfan syndrome?'

'Yes, he does. What did you make of his murmurs?'

'The systolic one was from the mitral valve, but it didn't sound like normal mitral regurgitation. I think the other one was aortic regurgitation.'

'It is and the mitral murmur isn't normal mitral regurge. It's mitral valve prolapse, which is due to

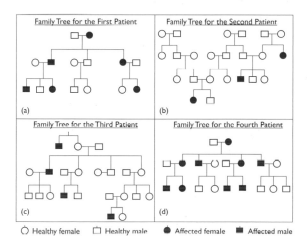

Family Tree for the First Patient	Family Tree for the Second Patient

Family Tree for the Third Patient	Family Tree for the Fourth Patient

○ Healthy female   □ Healthy male   ● Affected female   ■ Affected male

Figure 27.1 Four family trees showing different patterns of inheritance. See text for discussion.

ballooning of the cusps of the mitral valve. As for the aortic regurge, why should somebody with Marfan syndrome have that?'

'The same reason?'

'No, not quite. Patients with Marfan syndrome develop aneurysms of the thoracic aorta. If this dilates and distorts the root, the valve can become regurgitant. The cardiac abnormalities are a common and important cause of death. Do you know what the underlying abnormality is?'

Sarah shook her head.

'It's in one of a family of structural proteins, called fibrillins. The genes are on the long arm of chromosome 15.'

Dr Barrett discussed various aspects of the patient's condition with him, then showed Sarah the family tree for the next patient (Figure 27.1b).

'This one is autosomal recessive,' declared Sarah.

'Yes, it is. The patient needs to have two defective copies of the gene, so they often seem to be the first person in their family to be affected because the carriers tend not to manifest it. What sort of diseases tend to be autosomal recessive?'

'I'm sorry, I don't know, I hadn't thought of it like that before,' apologized Sarah.

'That's okay. It's typically diseases in which there's a defective enzyme or non-structural functional protein,

although there are exceptions, like with dominant inheritance. Most enzymes operate very efficiently and even if half the copies of an enzyme that a cell makes are defective, the other functioning half are normally enough to let the cell work properly. You need a double dose of the defective enzyme to produce symptoms. Why don't you take a history from this patient and her parents and come and tell me what you think the diagnosis is?'

Sarah obtained a history of a child who was born at term after a normal pregnancy. However, in the first few days, the child had bowel obstruction due to meconium ileus. Subsequently, there was a failure to grow at an appropriate rate despite a good diet and feeding. The child's stools were also offensive. A few years later, the child started to develop frequent chest infections.

'I think she's got cystic fibrosis,' offered Sarah.

'Very good,' said Dr Barrett. 'There are lots of different mutations that cause cystic fibrosis and they can produce different manifestations of the disease. They all affect a chloride ion channel on chromosome 7q. When this channel malfunctions various secretions become excessively viscous and cause blockages, especially in the pancreas and lungs. A lot of my work for this patient is going to be discussing the risks of her other siblings being carriers and the chances that if they are, they might

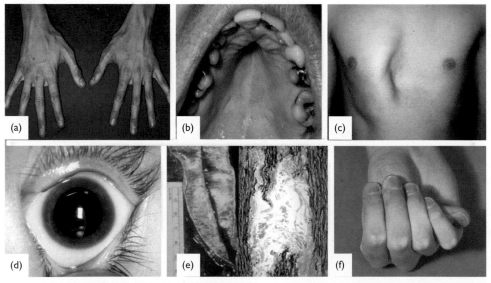

Figure 27.2 Some of the features of Marfan syndrome caused by defective fibrillin. (a) Arachnodactyly – long slender hands and feet; (b) high-arched palate with dental disarray; (c) pectus excavatum; (d) lax lens ligaments, allowing the lens to dislocate (this is usually in a 'down and out' direction, but the example shown here is 'down and in'); (e) aortic dissection, in which blood dissects along the media which contains weak elastic tissue (inset shows photomicrograph of the fragmented elastin); (f) Steinberg's sign – the thumb overhangs the edge of the hand when the fingers are closed over the thumb.

transmit the gene and what can be done to screen for it. The treatment for cystic fibrosis has improved a lot over the years, but it's still a very serious disease that significantly reduces life expectancy. Out of interest, do you know what group of people are most likely to be carriers?'

'No, not really.'

'White northern Europeans,' informed Dr Barrett. 'It's been suggested that being a carrier provided some resistance to cholera, which is why the gene was able to survive in the population at quite a high carrier prevalence. You should make sure that you're very familiar with cystic fibrosis before exam time.'

Given that Dr Barrett seemed to be arranging the cases in a logical order, Sarah had a pretty good idea what the next pattern of inheritance would be before she saw the family tree (Figure 27.1c).

'It's X-linked,' said Sarah, confidently.

'Dominant or recessive?' asked Dr Barrett, with a smile.

Sarah was caught off guard by this, but managed to gather her wits and deduced the answer. 'Recessive. The mothers must be carriers, but they don't have the disease.'

'Yep. There's no reason why a disease has to be recessive just because it's on the X chromosome. However, the odd thing is that almost all of them are. Now, if I were to tell you that this young boy bruises easily and has had trouble with bleeding into his joints, you'd probably be able to tell me the diagnosis.'

'Haemophilia.'

'Good. The other X-linked disease that people always think of is colour blindness, but there are quite a few more. Now, this next family tree might be a bit more difficult.'

Sarah had not been expecting a fourth type of inheritance. They had already done autosomal dominant and recessive diseases and X-linked conditions, so there didn't seem to be any other options left (Figure 27.1d).

'What do you see?' sought Dr Barrett, trying to coax the answer from Sarah.

'It's a large family. Different generations are affected, both male and female.'

'Mmm and what else? Where do all the children get the disease from?'

Sarah studied the family tree. 'None of the fathers have children who are affected,' she noticed. 'It's always the mothers who pass it on.'

'Absolutely. What type of DNA is only passed on by the mother?'

'Mitochondrial!' exclaimed Sarah, pleased with herself for having worked it out.

'That's it. The sperm's mitochondria are in its body and are left outside the egg when the head penetrates. Even if a few do sneak in, they're overwhelmed by the number of maternal mitochondria.'

'What sort of diseases are due to mitochondrial DNA?' asked Sarah.

'Not many, for a start. Those that are affect the nervous system, skeletal muscle and sometimes the heart. All the electrically excitable tissues that need to generate lots of energy to maintain their membrane potentials and/or contract. As one added thing, it's easy to forget that although mitochondria do have their own DNA, most of their proteins are actually coded on the nuclear DNA. Over time, it's believed that most of the mitochondrial genes got transferred to the nuclear DNA.

'So that's your four patterns of inheritance,' summarized Dr Barrett. 'There are subtleties like anticipation and co-dominant diseases, but we've covered the basics today, Sarah. Don't forget chromosomal diseases either. They can occasionally have an inherited component. Also don't forget that some people will just have a new spontaneous mutation so there won't be any family history at all.'

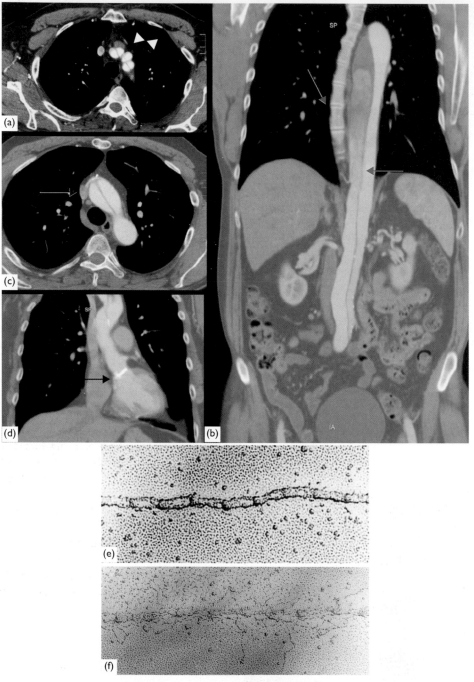

Figure 27.3 (a–d) CT scan image series in a 34-year-old man with Marfan syndrome which illustrates a life-threatening complication of the disease – aortic dissection; (e) SEM image of normal fibrillin ×40 000; (f) abnormal fibrillin ×46 000. Abnormal fibrillin causes weakness of the aortic wall, which can lead to blood leaking between the layers that make up the wall of the aorta. This can compromise the blood supply to major organs such as the brain, heart and abdominal organs. Rupture into the pericardial sac may occur, leading to fatal cardiac tamponade. The dissection raises an intimal flap which can be identified on cross-sectional imaging as a low-density line running through the origin of the brachiocephalic, carotid and subclavian arteries (white arrowhead), the aortic arch (red arrow) and the descending thoracic and abdominal aorta (green arrow). Note the aortic valve replacement (black arrow), a consequence of aortic regurgitation and the scoliosis of the thoracic spine (orange arrow) – all features of Marfan syndrome.

Sarah had almost completed her stint in the accident and emergency department and had enjoyed helping Dr Mike Costello, the senior A and E consultant. On an icy January evening, Harry, a 25-year-old electrician presented having slipped and fallen on his outstretched hand. Mike asked Sarah to go in and examine the patient's hand. Sarah found the young man holding his hand and wrist gingerly. The hand was swollen and tender particularly in the region of the anatomical snuff box.

Question 1

Where is the anatomical snuff box and why is it important?

Answer 1

The anatomical snuff box is a triangular-shaped concavity on the dorsal aspect of the hand between the thumb and index finger and along its radial aspect. In olden times, people who were fond of snorting snuff (tobacco) used to place the powder in this fossa and take a good sniff. Its importance for us lies in the fact that the scaphoid bone lies in the floor of the anatomical snuff box.

Scaphoid injuries are very common and in fact the scaphoid is the most commonly fractured carpal bone.

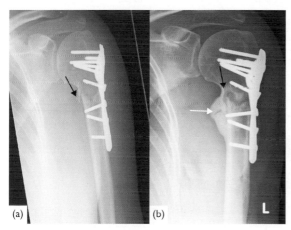

Figure 28.1 (a) Plating of a proximal humeral shaft fracture (arrow). (b) The fracture healing has occurred successfully with new bone at the margins of the fracture (periosteal callus – black arrow) and new bone bridging the fracture (endosteal callus – white arrow). For fracture healing to occur, reduction and immobilization are vital measures which the plate achieves.

Sarah told Mike she thought Harry had a scaphoid fracture. Mike agreed and sent the man off for some X-rays. Sarah felt a bit silly when the X-rays did not show a fracture. Mike smiled and reassured her. Scaphoid fractures are notorious for being hidden on X-rays, although well-taken radiographs should pick up most scaphoid fractures. Mike explained to Sarah that it is important to treat the patient as having a scaphoid fracture if there are clinical signs supporting this diagnosis until one can prove there is no fracture.

Question 2

What are the main principles of fracture management?

Answer 2

- Reduction – to restore bony alignment. This is important to allow the bone to heal back into its normal anatomical shape and position. If the bone does not heal in its normal shape or position it may not achieve its normal function and produce abnormal stresses on adjacent bones and joints. This can lead to arthritis in the joints and ongoing pain.
- Immobilization. This maintains alignment and allows healing to occur across the ends of the fractured bones without the process being interrupted by constant movement of the bone ends. Immobilization can be achieved with a plaster cast or with internal fixation through the use of screws, plates and pins. Splinting the bone also helps reduce the pain associated with the fracture.
- Rehabilitation. Over the period of immobilization muscles and bones become weak from disuse and may atrophy. Rehabilitation is aimed at restoring as much function and strength as possible after the fracture has healed.

Question 3

What may be the consequences of not recognizing and treating a scaphoid fracture?

Answer 3

Symptomatically the patient will suffer ongoing pain and loss of function with limited wrist motion and loss of grip strength. This would have devastating consequences for Harry, particularly if he couldn't grip a screwdriver! The structural consequences for the scaphoid may be more formally divided into:

- Malunion. The scaphoid does not heal in an anatomical position and shape. The abnormal shape predisposes to pain (with abnormal stresses on adjacent bones and joints) and loss of function.
- Non-union. The fracture fails to unite because of excessive movement at the fracture site. The fracture ends become covered with fibrocartilage and a false joint or pseudoarthrosis may result between the fragments.
- Delayed union. The fracture has not united completely after four months of immobilization. This usually occurs when there has been a significant delay in the diagnosis being made and treatment initiated.

- Arthritis. This occurs because of damage or excessive stress to the adjacent radiocarpal joint. Scaphoid fractures are also very commonly accompanied by damage to the carpal ligaments which contributes to eventual arthritic change.

The complications above can apply to fractures anywhere in the body. In addition, there may be:

- Avascular necrosis (AVN). AVN is a complication of fractures seen in only a few bones in the body – the scaphoid being one (it is also seen in the humeral and femoral head, talus and lunate bones). The proximal pole of the scaphoid does not have a direct blood supply and is fed from the waist of the scaphoid and the

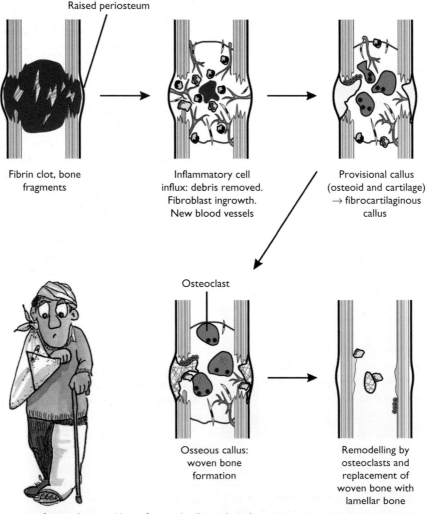

Raised periosteum

Fibrin clot, bone fragments

Inflammatory cell influx: debris removed. Fibroblast ingrowth. New blood vessels

Provisional callus (osteoid and cartilage) → fibrocartilaginous callus

Osteoclast

Osseous callus: woven bone formation

Remodelling by osteoclasts and replacement of woven bone with lamellar bone

Figure 28.2 The sequence of events in normal bone fracture healing and repair.

scaphoid tubercle distally. A fracture through the waist of the scaphoid may interrupt the blood supply leading to osteonecrosis of the proximal pole. AVN can occur even if the fracture is adequately treated and is dependent largely on where the fracture is. The proximal pole fragments over a period of time.

Question 4

Sarah followed Harry to the plaster room where the technician skilfully put a cast on Harry's wrist. Harry was given an appointment to come to the fracture clinic the next afternoon. The orthopaedic surgeon who saw Harry at the clinic sent him for an isotope bone scan to the radiology department. This was performed a week later and confirmed the presence of a scaphoid fracture. What are the options for imaging scaphoid fractures?

Answer 4

1. Isotope bone scan – the radioisotope injected is technetium-99 m diphosphonate, which is taken up by osteoblasts actively laying down new bone at fracture sites. Uptake may be seen at a scaphoid fracture site as early as two days after injury.
2. Plain films are repeated generally after a week and demonstrate the fracture line quite clearly. The fracture line becomes more conspicuous as bone fragments are resorbed by osteoclasts around the fracture.
3. CT (computed tomography) is used in some radiology departments to try and confirm the presence of a fracture but is mainly used to assess the position of fracture fragments if an operative repair is being considered.
4. MRI (magnetic resonance imaging) is being increasingly used in scaphoid injuries not only to demonstrate the fracture, but also to show associated ligamentous injuries and other occult bone fractures.

The optimal choice of imaging modality for diagnosing scaphoid fractures not seen on plain films is controversial and largely dictated by the ease of access to a particular imaging modality.

Question 5

How does a fractured bone heal?

Answer 5

At the fracture site, a kind of internal splint is formed by the haematoma, formed from clotted blood, and also

the localized tissue swelling, secondary to the release of inflammatory mediators. Polymorphs and macrophages from the blood and surrounding tissues appear within hours and increase in number over the next two days. They phagocytose the debris: bony fragments, blood clot and damaged connective tissue. Under the influence of inflammatory mediators, fibroblasts invade the wound site and the ingrowth of new capillaries is stimulated, carrying nutrients to the site. If pressed, the site is still slightly mobile at this stage, but is 'sticky', and is still tender. As the healing process progresses, fibrous tissue and cartilage is laid down, and this ossifies to form woven bone. This is the typical pattern of healing in a tubular long bone and will be modified slightly in other bone types.

At this point, the fracture is considered to be united, and is no longer tender or mobile under pressure, although it remains swollen. Several factors influence the rate at which fractures heal, particularly the type and site of the fracture (upper limbs heal quicker than lower, oblique or spiral fractures more quickly than transverse) and the age and nutritional state of the patient.

It will take several weeks or months more for the woven bone to be remodelled by osteoclasts within the bone, and for osteoblasts to lay down lamellar bone along the lines of stress, and the patient must be gently mobilized as soon as possible to assist this process. Once union has occurred and the patient is bearing weight, the lumpy new cortical bone gradually becomes resorbed and smoothed out and the excess medullary new bone is removed, restoring a normal medullary cavity. Woven bone, which is quite rapidly formed and which is much less efficient at weight bearing, is resorbed completely and is replaced by lamellar bone. This restoration to normality may take up to a year.

Harry had his cast removed after six weeks when his X-rays showed the fracture had healed. He then had several sessions with the hand physiotherapist trying to regain the strength in his wrist. He managed to get back to normal duties at work after three months.

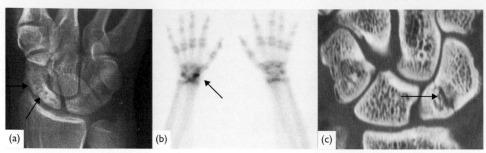

Figure 28.3 (a) Plain film showing a fracture through the waist of the scaphoid (thick arrow) with sclerosis of the proximal pole (thin arrow). This high density of the waist and proximal pole could be due to reversible ischaemia or irreversible avascular necrosis. (b) Technetium-99 m isotope bone scan showing osteoblastic uptake at the site of a scaphoid fracture in the right wrist (arrow). (c) Coronal CT showing a fracture through the proximal pole of the scaphoid (arrow).

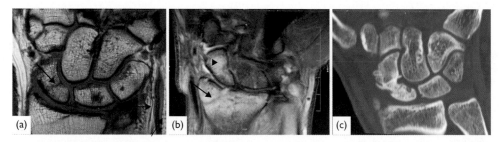

Figure 28.4 (a) T_1-weighted MRI – note the bright fatty marrow in the bones with a fracture line through the scaphoid (arrow). (b) Coronal T_2-weighted MRI with fat suppression showing a fracture through the radial styloid process (arrowhead) with high signal in the bone marrow indicating oedema. Note the bone marrow oedema involving the adjacent scaphoid, indicating microtrabecular injury which was occult on the plain films (arrow). (c) CT showing a contracted proximal pole of scaphoid which is sclerotic in keeping with avascular necrosis. This can be treated with bone grafting and internal fixation.

A 70-year-old woman, Mrs Moore, comes to casualty with severe back pain after stretching to open her bedroom window. On examination she is tender on palpation over her thoracolumbar junction.

Question 1

It is important to exclude 'sinister' features of back pain, what are these?

Answer 1

These include:

- alternating or bilateral sciatica
- weak legs
- weight loss or systemically unwell
- pyrexia of unknown origin (PUO) or raised erythrocyte sedimentation rate (ESR)
- history of neoplasia
- localized bony tenderness
- spine movement in all directions painful.

Question 2

What are the commonest causes of 'sinister' back pain?

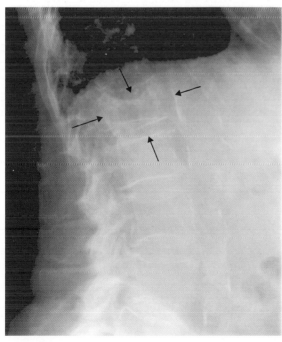

Figure 29.1 Lateral X-ray of the thoracolumbar spine showing loss in height of the L1 vertebral body with depression of the superior endplate (arrows).

Answer 2

- Bone metastases – most commonly from breast, bronchus, kidney and prostate cancers
- Myeloma
- Cord or paraspinal tumour
- Tuberculosis
- Abscess.

Question 3

Why is urgent treatment important and what may it involve?

Answer 3

There may be acute cord compression or acute cauda equina compression which can cause irreversible damage if not treated promptly.

Acute cauda equina compression gives:

- alternating or bilateral root pain in the legs
- saddle anaesthesia (bilateral around the anus)
- disturbance of bladder or bowel function.

Acute cord compression gives:

- bilateral pain
- lower motor neurone (LMN) signs at level of compression
- upper motor neurone (UMN) and sensory signs below the level of compression
- sphincter disturbance.

The treatment depends on the underlying lesion, so malignancies are likely to be treated by radiotherapy, abscesses will be decompressed and disc protrusions may have laminectomies.

Question 4

Mrs Moore has a lateral X-ray of her thoracolumbar spine (Figure 29.1). What does it show?

Answer 4

It shows loss in height of the L1 vertebral body with depression of the superior endplate. This is an osteoporotic crush fracture. Note the normal square shape of the vertebral bodies below. The bones are difficult to see and look 'rubbed out' – an appearance seen in osteoporosis.

Question 5

What do you understand by the terms 'pathological' fracture, 'stress' fracture, 'insufficiency' fracture and 'fatigue' fracture?

Answer 5

A pathological fracture is a break in bone which has been weakened by an underlying disease process such as tumour, infection, inherited bone disorders, Paget's disease and osteoporosis. The term 'stress' fracture is used to describe a fracture which results from submaximal forces over a period of time. Stress fractures are subdivided into 'insufficiency' and 'fatigue' fractures. Insufficiency fractures are a type of pathological fracture in which normal forces produce a fracture in weakened bone. Fatigue fractures result from repeated abnormal stresses to normal bone, e.g. march fractures

of the metatarsal bones in marching infantry or marathon runners.

Question 6

What is osteoporosis?

Answer 6

Osteoporosis occurs when bone becomes demineralized faster than the body can replace the minerals. Bones become fragile and weak and may break with normal stresses, such as climbing stairs and opening windows. Sites susceptible to osteoporotic fractures include the distal radius (the Colles' fracture), the pelvis, femoral neck and vertebral column. The condition is very common in the elderly affecting almost 80 per cent of postmenopausal women. Osteoporotic patients gradually lose height over time as they develop crush fractures in several vertebrae. The back also

Squares in the graphs (right) indicate patient's densitometry is 4 S.D. below that of a young adult and has not changed from previous reading.

Region	BMD (g/cm²)	Young-Adult T-Score	Age-Matched Z-Score
L1	0.634	−4.1	−3.8
L2	0.683	−4.3	−4.0
L3	0.788	−3.4	−3.1
L4	0.650	−4.6	−4.3
L1–L3	0.710	−3.8	−3.5
L1–L4	0.692	−4.1	−3.8
L2–L3	0.739	−3.8	−3.5
L2–L4	0.706	−4.1	−3.8

		Trend: L2–L4	Change vs	
Measured Date	Age (years)	BMD (g/cm²)	Previous (%)	Previous (g/cm²)
17/04/2007	55.5	0.706	–	–

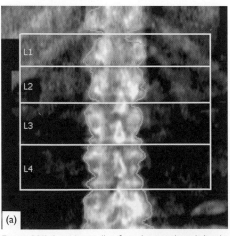

(a)

(b)

Figure 29.2 Sample reading from bone mineral densitometry (BMD) (see p. 114 for discussion).

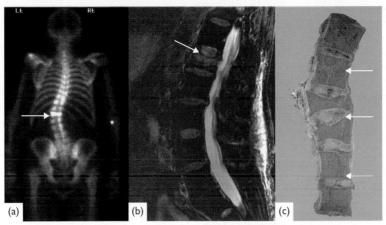

Figure 29.3 (a) Isotope bone scan showing activity in the L1 vertebral fracture (arrow) indicating that there is an osteoblastic response at the fracture site and also indirectly indicating that this is a relatively recent and symptomatic injury. This is helpful if there is doubt about whether the fracture is new or old and also in determining if there is an occult fracture elsewhere in the vertebral column which may be the symptomatic lesion. (b) Sagittal short TI inversion recovery (STIR) MRI showing bone marrow oedema in the L1 crush fracture (arrow). The bright signal reflects increased water content at the fracture site. This tells the radiologist this is an acute and symptomatic injury which may benefit from vertebroplasty. (c) Typical appearance of a pathological wedge fracture of vertebra (red arrow). In this example the spine contains metastatic tumour (black arrows).

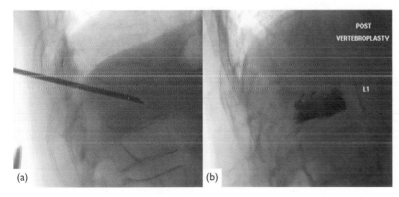

Figure 29.4 (a) Vertebroplasty showing the needle going through a pedicle into the L1 vertebral body. (b) Post-vertebroplasty image showing cement successfully injected into the body.

becomes more curved (kyphotic) as the vertebrae become wedged.

Question 7

What are the risk factors for osteoporosis?

Answer 7

- Menopause – lack of oestrogen leads to rapid demineralization of bone
- Decreased calcium and vitamin intake
- Inactive lifestyle
- Alcohol
- Smoking.

This is often referred to as primary osteoporosis

Question 8

What is secondary osteoporosis?

Answer 8

Secondary osteoporosis is when certain conditions and treatments predispose individuals to osteoporosis, such as:

- rheumatoid arthritis
- chronic liver disease
- chronic renal failure
- malabsorption syndromes – e.g. Crohn's disease, coeliac disease
- hyperthyroidism

- hyperparathyroidism
- long-term steroids.

Osteoporosis can be diagnosed by the appearance of the bone on plain films and by assessment of bone mineral density (BMD). Conventionally, the mean BMD is assessed over the region of bone from L2 to L4 and the mean is compared with that expected in a young adult reference population aged 20–45 of the same sex (the t- score). A mean reading that is 2.5 standard deviations below the reference mean or less (i.e. t-score <2.5) is regarded as osteoporotic by World Health Organization criteria (Figure 29.2).

Question 9

Osteoporotic crush fractures of the spine have been treated in the past with prolonged bed rest and analgesia. What are the risks of prolonged bed rest and analgesia in the elderly?

Answer 9

- Thromboembolic disease (deep vein thrombosis and pulmonary embolism)
- Gastrointestinal irritation (from NSAIDs and opiates)
- Pneumonia.

Question 10

Our patient is referred by the admitting orthopaedic team to the radiology department for consideration of percutaneous therapy to try and relieve the patient's symptoms. What procedure are they going to perform and what does it involve?

Answer 10

Vertebroplasty is a procedure performed by interventional radiologists and some orthopaedic surgeons under fluoroscopic guidance. Basically the procedure involves the injection of orthopaedic 'cement' into the crush fracture. The idea is to stabilize the vertebral body. Many patients get instant relief of their pain after the procedure. Many patients get back home and regain function within a week or two following vertebroplasty. Further collapse of the vertebra is prevented. The procedure is performed with sedation and the patient lying on their stomach on the X-ray table. A large needle is pushed through the pedicle of the involved vertebra into the body and cement is slowly injected. The radiologist monitors the flow of cement into the body on the fluoroscopy screen.

There are risks inherent in the procedure. The cement may enter the disc space (increasing the chance of a fracture in the adjacent vertebra), intraosseous veins (with the risk of embolization) and into the spinal canal (with a risk of paraplegia). There is a lack of controlled trials assessing bed rest versus vertebroplasty. There is, however, no doubt that some patients regain function and become asymptomatic remarkably quickly after this procedure.

A 42-year-old man presents to the accident and emergency department after a grand mal seizure having had a headache and feeling unwell for several weeks. He is a little confused and has a slight weakness with brisk reflexes in the right arm and leg. He has an extensor plantar response in his right foot. He has a subtle facial weakness on his right side affecting predominantly the lower part of his face. His wife has noticed he has had trouble sometimes understanding what she is saying in the last few weeks.

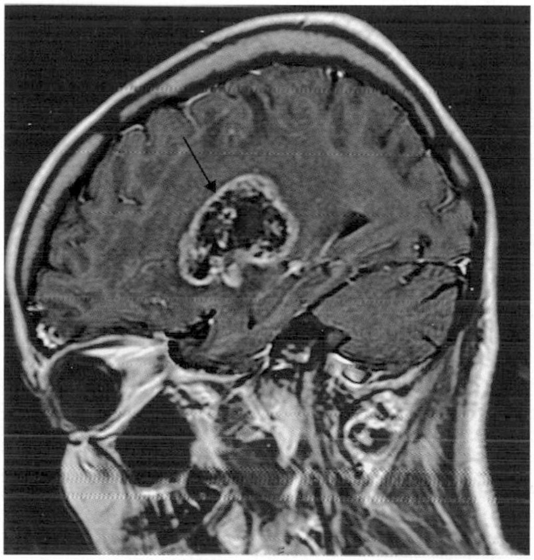

Question 1

Where do you think the lesion responsible for the man's presentation lies anatomically?

Answer 1

The brisk reflexes and motor weakness affecting the right side of his body and face suggest a lesion that involves the pyramidal tracts originating in the left motor cortex. The facial muscles in the upper part of the face are supplied by motor tracts arising from both sides of the cerebral hemisphere so therefore a unilateral lesion above the level of the facial nerve nucleus in the brain stem results in weakness predominantly of the lower part of the face (a unilateral lesion involving the facial nerve or its nucleus therefore results in weakness of one side of the face both in the upper and lower parts). Disorders of the comprehension and formulation of speech are termed dysphasias and are discussed in Case 12, Permanent neurological signs (p. 44).

The combination of signs and symptoms suggest a lesion high in the left cerebral hemisphere.

Question 2

What does the length of the history tell you about the likely underlying process?

Answer 2

This is a slightly more difficult question as the patient has both insidious and acute symptoms. An

Figure 30.1 The MRI shows a solitary irregular lesion in the brain with ring enhancement. Enhancement implies a disturbance of the blood–brain barrier. There are non-enhancing cystic/necrotic components. This is characteristic of a high-grade neoplasm arising from the glial constituents of the brain – a glioblastoma multiforme (arrow).

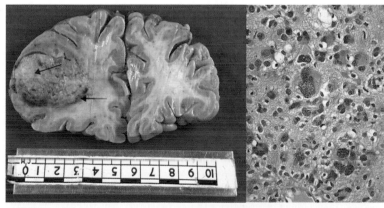

(a)   (b)

Figure 30.2 (a) Coronal slice of brain showing a glioblastoma multiforme. The aggressive nature of this tumour can be inferred from the presence of widespread necrosis (red arrow) and haemorrhage (blue arrow) and the irregular border of the tumour. These lesions sometimes extend across the midline of the brain in a 'butterfly' distribution. (b) Microscopy shows highly pleomorphic malignant astrocytes (H&E medium power).

acute neurological dysfunction – a stroke – arises from a lesion that has rapidly evolved, usually an infarct or a cerebral bleed. Lesions with a more insidious course have grown slightly more slowly (e.g. an abscess or a tumour). Plaques of demyelination can sit on both sides of the acute and insidious fence. The seizure is the acute symptom and suggests irritation of neurons resulting in a temporary excessive neuronal discharge.

The patient went on to have a CT and MRI study. The MRI study showed a solitary irregular lesion in the left hemisphere with some patchy enhancement (Figure 30.1). The enhancement means there is a disturbance of the blood–brain barrier. The lesion has some non-enhancing cystic components and exerts mass effect on the surrounding brain. This is characteristic of a high grade neoplasm arising from the glial constituents of the brain – a glioblastoma multiforme (GBM).

Sometimes a solitary metastasis can have a similar appearance and presentation but usually there are multiple lesions and in the course of investigation we usually uncover a primary in the lung, breast, colon or a melanoma.

Question 3

What does the grading of a brain tumour imply?

Answer 3

Tumour grading indicates the degree of similarity to normal brain cells. Any particular brain tumour can have low-, mid- and high-grade tumour cells – the most malignant cell usually determines the grade. The grading of a brain tumour influences its treatment and the overall prognosis for the patient.

The World Health Organization has been working on the grading and description of brain tumours for at least 30 years. Their most recent classification assigns a numerical grade to brain tumours reflecting their degree of malignancy from an ascending scale of I (benign) to IV (highly malignant).

Question 4

Describe the various types of brain tumours.

Answer 4

As with tumours elsewhere, it is best to think about the tissues present and what they can give rise to. This gives us a list of tumours:

- Neuroglia
  - astrocytomas including the high-grade glioblastoma multiforme
  - oligodendrogliomas
  - ependymomas
  - choroid plexus papillomas
- Neurons
  - neuroblastoma and ganglioneuroma
- Meninges
  - meningioma
- Nerve sheath
  - schwannoma and neurofibroma
- Embryonal
  - primitive neuro-ectodermal tumours
- Other
  - primary CNS lymphoma, germ cell tumours, craniopharyngiomas and, of course, metastatic tumours.

The list is not exhaustive and definitive diagnosis requires biopsy.

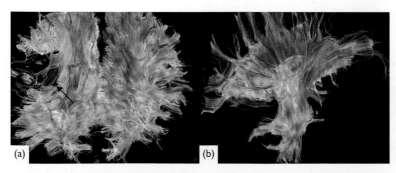

Figure 30.3 MR tractography. (a) Coronal slice in our patient showing the interruption of the white matter tracts by the glioblastoma multiforme (arrow). (b) Sagittal section in the same patient showing normal white matter tracts in the right hemisphere.

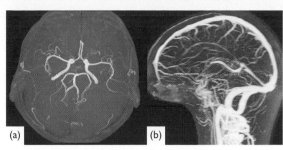

Figure 30.4 (a) MR arteriography showing the circle of Willis at the base of the brain. (b) MR venography showing the dural venous drainage of the brain.

Question 5

What other conditions can mimic brain tumours clinically?

Answer 5

Any condition causing a space-occupying lesion can present in a similar way, for example, an aneurysm, abscess, chronic subdural haematoma or cysts.

Our unfortunate patient was referred to the neurosurgeons and had a palliative resection followed by radiotherapy and chemotherapy. It is very difficult to completely resect and treat a GBM because the tumour infiltrates white matter tracts more extensively than is represented by the lesion we see on imaging and the surgeon sees on the operating table.

Question 6

What are the best imaging techniques to use?

Answer 6

MRI has a major role in the assessment of brain tumours and their suitability for surgery. It can hint at the grade of tumour – a high-grade tumour tends to be more heterogeneous, have more mass effect and demonstrate more enhancement.

Ancillary imaging techniques include:

- Spectroscopy. This uses MRI to assess the distribution of metabolites in a volume of tissue. Brain tumours tend to have a particular distribution of metabolites which differs from normal brain tissue.
- MR/CT perfusion. This looks at qualitative as well as quantitative aspects of cerebral blood flow. Higher grade brain tumours show more perfusion than normal brain.
- Tractography (Figure 30.3). This uses special MR techniques to map out the white matter tracts in the brain. This is becoming useful as surgeons will be able to work out which white matter tracts are affected by the tumour and are likely to be affected by their surgery.

MR arteriography and venography map out the cerebral arteries and major draining dural veins.

Sarah McKenzie had visited the mortuary a few times before to watch post mortems but this was the first occasion on which she was viewing an autopsy on a patient she had known herself.

Sarah was accompanied by Mr Quested, the plastic surgeon who had been closely involved in the treatment of the deceased, John Markham, a 25-year-old tree surgeon.

A few other medical students joined Sarah and Mr Quested in the viewing gallery of the mortuary, as did some members of Mr Quested's team.

A series of trays were laid out by the glass partition that separated the viewing gallery from the dissecting area of the mortuary. Wet blue paper towels covered the contents of the trays.

Two minutes after Sarah and Mr Quested arrived, the pathologist, Bob Austin, emerged from the door that led from the dissecting area into the changing rooms. Despite a name that made him sound close to retirement, Dr Austin was still the low side of 40.

'Is everybody here?' asked Dr Austin. Sarah recognized him from her previous visits to the mortuary.

Mr Quested answered in the affirmative. 'Would you like to present the case, Sarah?' he asked.

Sarah knew that Mr Quested wanted her to summarize the history. She had been in the plastic surgery outpatient clinic when Mr Markham had first presented a little over a year ago and had been able to follow his case through his first excision, subsequent operations and other admissions up until his death two days ago.

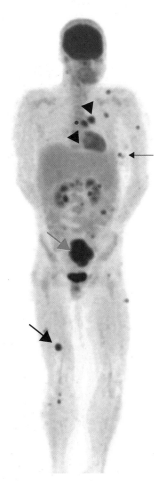

Figure 31.2 Whole-body PET scan in a 20-year-old patient with metastatic melanoma. Positron emission tomography (PET), a nuclear medicine imaging technique, uses fluorine-18 fluorodeoxyglucose (FDG), a radioisotope which is a glucose analogue taken up by metabolically active tissue. The PET scan detects areas of very high metabolic activity such as brain, muscle, brown fat, but also most cancers. PET is increasingly used for staging malignancies and assessing treatment response. This scan shows multiple metastatic deposits, including subcutaneous deposits in the left breast (thin black arrow), a deposit in the femur (red arrow), a pelvic uterine metastasis (green arrow) and multiple hilar, mediastinal and mesenteric lymph node deposits (arrowheads).

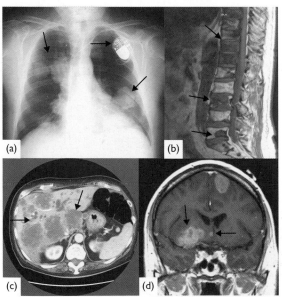

Figure 31.1 (a) Chest X-ray showing 'cannon ball' metastases in the lungs (arrows). (b) Sagittal MRI showing multiple spinal metastases (arrows). (c) Axial post-contrast CT showing multiple liver metastases (arrows). (d) Coronal MRI showing multiple metastases in the brain (arrows).

'Mr Markham was a 25-year-old man who presented to Mr Quested's clinic one year ago with a pigmented lesion on his back,' began Sarah, giving the presentation she had prepared of a history that was already familiar to her and one that she could have related without any practice. 'It had been noticed by his new girlfriend four weeks before the clinic. The mole was about the size of a 10p piece and had an irregular outline, irregular pigmentation and was a bit lumpy. Mr Markham knew he had a mole at that site, but as far as he was aware it should have been a lot smaller, flat and uniform, so this suggested that the mole had changed.'

Bob Austin nodded. 'Did it have any other sinister features?' he asked.

'No. It wasn't bleeding or itching.'

'Okay, sorry to interrupt, I just wanted to bring that out for the benefit of your colleagues,' explained Dr Austin, nodding at the other students. 'Worrying moles are those that change, bleed, itch or are irregular in outline, pigmentation or contour.'

Sarah resumed her presentation. 'Mr Markham had an excision biopsy a week later. The pathology report showed that it was a superficial spreading melanoma, in

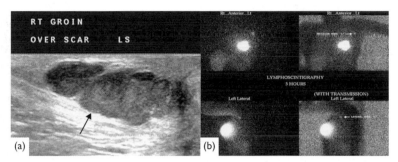

Figure 31.3 (a) Ultrasound showing a melanoma-containing lymph node (arrow) in the groin. Ultrasound guidance is used by radiologists to obtain fine needle aspiration cytology (FNAC) of these lesions to confirm the diagnosis of metastatic melanoma. (b) The sentinel node is the first lymph node that drains a tumour, so this is the first node that will develop a metastasis. If this node is removed and histologically does not contain tumour then theoretically the other nodes will not contain metastatic deposits, therefore the patient will not require an extensive lymph node dissection (which can cause several complications). Preoperatively, circumferential peritumoral transdermal injections of technetium-99 m antimony colloid are made. Imaging with a gamma camera is commenced. Uptake in the sentinel node is sometimes demonstrated within minutes. The node (arrow) is marked with a skin marker and is then removed in theatre using both the marker and a radioactive detector.

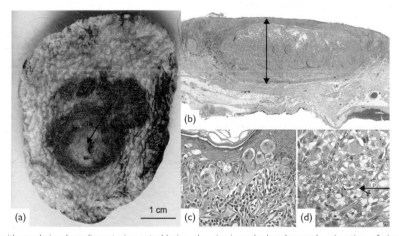

Figure 31.4 (a) Skin with an obviously malignant pigmented lesion, showing irregular borders and variegation of pigmentation. The arrowed area is in vertical growth phase. (b) Low-power microscopy shows melanoma with a Breslow depth of 4.6 mm (arrow), Clark level 3 (deep dermis). The arrowed area is in vertical growth phase. (c) Adjacent superficial spreading melanoma at medium magnification, with intraepidermal nests of tumour cells, and invasive tumour in horizontal growth phase is seen on either side of the nodular mass. (d) High-power view from the nodular area shows malignant cytological features such as pleomorphic cells and an atypical quadripolar mitotic figure (arrow).

vertical growth phase, with a Breslow thickness of 2.9 mm, a Clark level of 4, a mitotic count of 2 per square millimetre, without evidence of regression and without ulceration.'

'Clearly you know your stuff, Sarah,' complimented Dr Austin. 'Again, for the benefit of your colleagues, those are the key prognostic parameters of a melanoma. The two most important are the Breslow thickness and the growth phase. A melanoma can either be in horizontal or vertical growth phase. Horizontal phase melanomas tend to grow sideways but don't invade down deeply. Vertical growth phase melanomas are considered to have the ability to penetrate deeply and behave more aggressively. That's considered to be a bad feature because deep in the dermis is where the bigger blood vessels and lymphatics are that provide a metastatic route for the tumour. The Breslow thickness is a measure of the depth of invasion. The larger the Breslow, the worse the prognosis, for a similar reason. Thicker tumours are more likely to have found a way to break out of the primary site and metastasize and once a malignant tumour starts to do that, it's typically bad news.'

'As is normal treatment, a wide local excision of the scar was planned. Because Mr Markham's melanoma was in vertical growth phase and was thick enough, he also needed a sentinel node biopsy,' continued Sarah.

'And what's the rationale behind that, Sarah?' inquired Mr Quested.

Sarah had not known much about sentinel node theory before meeting Mr Markham, but the question did not now pose any difficulties for her. 'The idea is that a tumour site drains through a particular set of lymphatic channels. If you can find out where the first lymph node along those channels is and you can take that node out, you can see if the tumour has spread. If the lymph node is negative, it's likely that you've caught the tumour before it's had a chance to disseminate by the lymphatics. If it's positive then you would aim to resect all of the lymph nodes in that region to try to clear the metastases while they're still making their way through the lymph node complex. People whose sentinel lymph nodes are clear have a better prognosis.'

'Are there any other cancers where this technique is also used?'

'Breast and penile.'

'Excellent. Go on.'

'Mr Markham's sentinel lymph node was in his left axilla and was positive,' continued Sarah. 'He had an axillary lymph node dissection and there was tumour in 9 out of 24 lymph nodes. He remained well for four months, then developed a nodule on his anterior chest, which turned out to be a subcutaneous metastasis. Over the next four months he had several more cutaneous metastases. A month after the last of these was removed, he started to pass dark, tarry, black stools. An OGD [oesophagogastroduodenoscopy] found an ulcerated lesion in the duodenum that turned out to be melanoma. A CT scan showed pulmonary and liver metastases. There were no medical oncological options available other than supportive care and surgical resection wasn't possible. He deteriorated slowly and died two days ago.'

'That's very comprehensive, thank you, Sarah,' said Dr Austin. 'Starting with the external examination, there were scars that were compatible with the assorted previous operations.'

Dr Austin removed the wet tissue paper from the trays to reveal a set of dissected organs. 'The heart you can see here was normal, as was the aorta. There are a few fatty streaks but really very minimal atheroma. The heart's normally not thought of as a site for metastases, but melanoma is one of the tumours that is more likely to go there, but not in this patient's case.

'These are the lungs, the right one here and the left one next to it. There are multiple nodules of various sizes scattered throughout both lungs. Some of them are necrotic, other show some pigmentation. Not all melanomas produce significant amounts of melanin and not all that do continue to when they spread and conversely, not everything that's pigmented is a melanoma, but in this case, it's a useful feature in the context.

'The oesophagus and stomach are normal. The small bowel shows six ulcerated tumours. These are widely separated and trying to excise these while leaving enough bowel for adequate absorption would have been challenging at best. The colon's holding its own, although that's of limited consolation.

'You can see that liver's got lots of mets in it. The LFTs [liver function tests] were normal, but that's not too surprising. The liver can absorb a remarkable volume of metastases and still maintain adequate function, as gauged by LFTs. The gallbladder's minding its own business, as are the pancreas and spleen.

'The kidneys were thought to be normal, but there's actually a metastasis in the upper pole of the right kidney. Like the heart, the kidneys aren't commonly cited as a place for metastases. It has been suggested that they're relatively resistant, but nobody's told melanomas that because they'll quite happily go to the kidney. Lymphomas and leukaemias also manage to bypass any defences the kidney may have.

'The ureters, bladder and prostate are normal.

'The adrenals and thyroid gland are also normal.

'That just leaves the brain. I couldn't find anything in the notes to suggest an intracranial lesion, but he's got a small met in his left frontal lobe here and one in the posterior right parietal lobe. They're small and wouldn't have produced a big enough mass effect to give a midline shift and it looks like they missed any areas that would cause a recognizable focal syndrome.

'So, in summary, we've got a 25-year-old man with evidence of metastatic melanoma in multiple organs. I'll be taking some histology to confirm that they're melanomas, but I don't anticipate any surprises.'

'That's great, thanks, Bob,' said Mr Quested.

'There's another question for the students to be thinking about,' added Dr Austin. 'We've seen the ability of a malignant tumour to metastasize, but what properties does a tumour need to have to allow it to do that?'

The discussion around this question went on for several minutes, but Sarah and the other students managed to establish the following points. Metastasis is complex and requires numerous properties of the tumour:

- Ability to move.
- Detachment from adjacent cells (loss of cell–cell adhesion molecules) to take advantage of any movement capability.
- Invasion, which requires the breakdown of basement membranes and the extracellular matrix (including collagenases, metallomatrix proteases and plasminogen activator).
- Survival away from the comfort of the normal environment to which the cell of origin would have been adapted.
- Angiogenesis to provide a vascular supply. The metastasis needs a network of blood vessels to support its growth.
- Avoiding elimination by the immune system. The immune system can recognize some nascent neoplastic cells as foreign and destroy them.
- Ability to enter lymphatic and blood vessels. The tumour has to be able to spread from the primary site and these are excellent routes.
- Survival in the lymphovascular system. Entering the lymphovascular system is no guarantee that the detached cells can survive there.
- Attachment to endothelial cells and exiting the vessel.
- Ability to infiltrate foreign tissue and survive in a new cellular environment.

Jack is a healthy, happy baby born three months earlier at full term to Kylie. Kylie is 17 and lives with her mother and one younger sibling in a small flat. Kylie and her family dote on Jack, who really loves all the attention, but for the last 36 hours he has been a little unwell with a snuffly nose and not really being interested in feeding. Kylie is concerned because Jack is her first baby, but her mother reassures her that this is nothing unusual. Jack is settled down for the night, lying on his back just as Kylie has been taught at her mother and baby classes and sleeping in a cot in Kylie's room. At six o'clock, Kylie wakes and looks over at Jack. Something doesn't seem quite right. She goes over to pick him up and he is cool and not breathing. She shouts for her mother, an ambulance is called, resuscitation is attempted but there is no sign of life. Jack is dead.

Question 1

What are the most common causes of death in a three-month-old child?

Answer 1

In a child who was born at term without any complications, the most common causes of death will be 'cot deaths' (SIDS = sudden infant death syndrome), infection and undiagnosed congenital anomalies, especially cardiac defects. An uncommon but important cause, with implications for other members of the family, is inborn errors of metabolism. Infant deaths are more common if mothers are under 20 years of age or older than 40 years. Teenage mothers are particularly likely to have a baby who suffers a cot death, whereas older mothers have babies with greater risk of congenital anomalies.

Question 2

What investigations should be performed in the accident and emergency department immediately after death?

Answer 2

The infant should be carefully examined by a consultant looking especially for skin marks, abrasions and discoloration, which should be photographed by a police photographer if deemed significant. This is because colour changes due to local pressure (e.g. around the nose or neck) may fade before the autopsy. With the permission of the coroner (generally given as part of the locally agreed procedure for handling these cases) the samples

Table 32.1 Samples to be taken immediately after death

Blood:	Toxicology
	Aerobic and anaerobic culture
	Cytogenetics (if dysmorphic)
	Inherited metabolic diseases (use Guthrie card)
Nasopharyngeal aspirate:	Bacterial and viral studies
CSF:	Microscopy and culture
Urine:	Toxicology and inherited Metabolic diseases
Swabs from any lesions:	Culture
Possible additional tests:	Skin fibroblast cultures
	Muscle biopsy if mitochondrial disorder suspected

NB: For legal reasons it is important to ensure an unbroken 'chain of evidence' when taking samples and delivering them to the laboratory.

listed in Table 32.1 should be obtained; if not already taken as part of the resuscitation process.

Note: For legal reasons, it is important to ensure an unbroken 'chain of evidence' when taking samples and delivering them to the laboratory.

Question 3

What is the role of the police or coroner's officers in these circumstances?

Answer 3

Within 24 hours of the death, a specially trained police officer working with a paediatrician should visit the bereaved family at home so that they can see the sleeping arrangements and the family can explain what happened. Most deaths at this age will be natural, but a minority are a consequence of ignorance, neglect or abuse. The combined skills of a health professional and a police officer are best suited to extract the relevant evidence.

Question 4

What is the purpose of the autopsy?

Answer 4

The autopsy looks for natural causes of death and also aims to identify any unnatural or suspicious features.

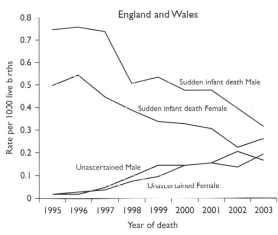

Figure 32.1 Rates for sudden infant death declined from the mid-1990s and this coincided with a campaign to put babies to sleep on their backs. (Redrawn from data in www.statistics.gov.uk/articles/hsq/HSQ27infant_death.pdf. Crown copyright material is reproduced with the permission of the Controller of HMSO and the Queen's Printer for Scotland.)

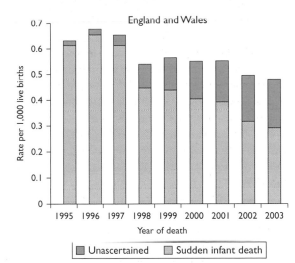

Figure 32.2 The decrease in rates for sudden infant deaths coincided with an increase in 'unascertained deaths', suggesting that a part of the decline could be due to changes in classification. This means that it can be helpful to consider both categories together (as in Figures 32.2 and 32.3). (Redrawn from data in www.statistics.gov.uk/articles/hsq/HSQ27infant_death.pdf. Crown copyright material is reproduced with the permission of the Controller of HMSO and the Queen's Printer for Scotland.)

It should be performed by a pathologist with a specialist interest in paediatric pathology who is familiar with the conditions that can manifest in the first year of life. They need to have access to the information gleaned from the home visit with the parents. Often the home-visit police officer will attend the autopsy. If the pathologist discovers any suspicious features then they will usually involve a forensic pathologist.

Question 5

What are the standard investigations at autopsy?

Answer 5

Before the autopsy commences, there should be a full skeletal survey reported by a paediatric radiologist to look for evidence of recent or old trauma. The autopsy involves a detailed external examination to assess growth, nutrition, hydration, any dysmorphic features and to look for natural or unnatural surface lesions. The internal examination involves detailed dissection to search for anatomical abnormalities, inspection of all organs and tissues and the taking of samples for histological, microbiological and biochemical investigations. In all cases of unexplained, unexpected deaths, frozen sections are performed for fat staining on liver and kidney as a screening test for a broad range of metabolic problems.

Question 6

What additional investigations may be needed?

Answer 6

If the history raises the possibility of drug or alcohol ingestion, then a toxicology screen on blood, urine and stomach contents is indicated. If the fat staining or other evidence suggests a metabolic problem, then bile and blood on Guthrie cards for acylcarnitine studies are important. If a genetic anomaly is suspected, then skin for fibroblast culture and liver or other solid organ for DNA extraction may be useful.

Question 7

How are sudden deaths in infancy classified?

Answer 7

If the death has a specific natural cause, such as congenital heart disease or pneumonia, then that will be the cause of death. SIDS is the sudden and unexpected death of an apparently healthy infant, whose death remains unexplained after the performance of an adequate investigation including an autopsy, investigation

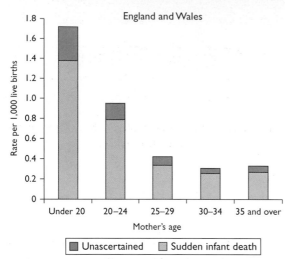

England and Wales

Figure 32.3 Young mothers are most likely to suffer a sudden infant death. (Redrawn from data in www.statistics.gov.uk/articles/hsq/HSQ27infant_death.pdf. Crown copyright material is reproduced with the permission of the Controller of HMSO and the Queen's Printer for Scotland.)

often inferred to mean suspicious but unproven. Families may feel there is stigma associated with this category so coroners are advised not to use this unnecessarily as the final cause of death. Immediately after performing an autopsy which does not reveal an obvious natural cause, the pathologist will conclude 'unexplained pending further investigation'.

Question 8

Who looks after the family?

Answer 8

Babies found dead at home should go to the accident and emergency department and not directly to a mortuary. The family should be allocated a member of staff to look after them and a consultant paediatrician should be involved, who should explain that their child has died, how the police and coroner will be involved and the requirement for an autopsy. After the autopsy, the SUDI doctor or another health professional should discuss the results with the parents (provided that it is not a suspicious death).

The multi-agency protocol requires all the professionals to meet to discuss the case after the home visit and autopsy so as to provide a report for the coroner, a detailed letter for the family and a plan of further support for the family. There are also various charities, such as FSID (Foundation for the Study of Infant Deaths), who can provide advice and support.*

of the scene and circumstances of the death, and exploration of the medical history of the infant and family.

If a sudden death does not meet these international criteria for SIDS (most commonly because of inadequate information and investigation), then it should be classified as SUDI (sudden unexpected death in infancy). There is a category of 'unascertained' that is

*The answers in this case are based on the report of a working group convened by the Royal College of Pathologists and the Royal College of Paediatrics and Child Health (2004) entitled 'Sudden Unexpected Death in Infancy – A multi-agency protocol for care and investigation'. This is based on the legal system for England and Wales.

A 68-year-old man consults his GP because he has noticed a yellowish discoloration of his skin and sclerae that has developed over the previous few weeks. Examination confirms the presence of jaundice.

Question 1

What is jaundice?

Answer 1

Jaundice can be defined purely on biochemical terms as being an elevated level of bilirubin in the blood. However, it is more often used to indicate a yellowish discoloration of the sclerae and/or skin that is due to a raised bilirubin.

Jaundice may be either a sign or a symptom.

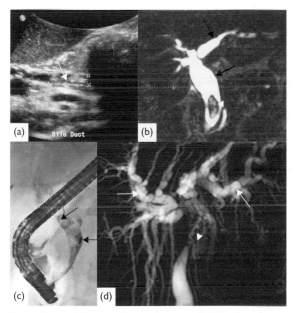

Figure 33.1 (a) Ultrasound image showing gallstones (arrow) in the common bile duct. (b) MR cholangiopancreatography (MRCP) showing dilated bile ducts (thin black arrows) with a gallstone (white arrowhead) impacted in the common bile duct. (c) Endoscopic retrograde cholaniopancreatography (ERCP) showing multiple gallstones as filling defects (arrows) in the common bile duct. (d) MRCP showing a stricture of the common hepatic duct and common bile duct (arrowhead) with marked dilation of the intrahepatic ducts (white arrows). This is caused by a malignancy of the bile ducts – a cholangiocarcinoma.

Question 2

Where is jaundice first likely to be noticed?

Answer 2

The sclerae of the eyes are typically the first part of the body to exhibit discernible jaundice.

Question 3

What is the source of the pigment in jaundice?

Answer 3

The bilirubin that causes the yellow pigmentation in jaundice is a breakdown product of haem and is therefore mainly derived from haemoglobin in erythrocytes; a smaller amount is generated by the degradation of myoglobin.

Question 4

How is bilirubin metabolized?

Answer 4

Bilirubin is derived from haem and this occurs when old erythrocytes undergo destruction in the spleen and other parts of the reticuloendothelial system. This bilirubin is initially bound to albumin and is transported to the liver where is undergoes glucuronidation. This makes the bilirubin more water soluble and facilitates its excretion into the duodenum in bile.

Once in the gastrointestinal tract, bacterial action converts conjugated bilirubin into urobilinogen, most of which is oxidised to urobilin. The bulk of the urobilinogen and urobilin are excreted in the faeces, but some of the urobilinogen is reabsorbed in the small bowel and is then excreted by the kidney.

Question 5

What are the causes of jaundice?

Answer 5

Many metabolic derangements, such as jaundice, disturbances of glucose and electrolyte imbalances, can be considered using a fairly simple framework:

- Increased levels are caused by increased intake or production, altered metabolism or distribution, decreased excretion.

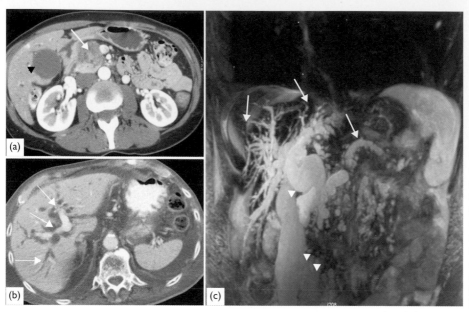

Figure 33.2 (a) CT showing a mass in the head of the pancreas (arrow) with a distended gallbladder (arrowhead). (b) CT showing dilated intrahepatic ducts (arrows). (c) Three-dimensional MR cholangiopancreatography showing gross dilation of the common bile duct (arrowhead), intrahepatic ducts and pancreatic duct (white arrows) with a malignant stricture of the distal common bile duct (double arrowhead) due to a carcinoma of the head of the pancreas.

- Decreased levels are caused by decreased intake or production, altered metabolism or distribution, increased excretion.

In very simple terms, this may be thought of as 'in, out, shake it all about'.

For jaundice, this system becomes pre-hepatic, hepatic and post-hepatic.

- Pre-hepatic jaundice can arise if the production of bilirubin exceeds the capacity of the liver to metabolize it. The rate-limiting step in the handling of bilirubin by the liver is the excretion of conjugated bilirubin to the bile canaliculi, rather than the conjugation reaction itself. As the normal daily load of bilirubin is only one-tenth of the liver's total bilirubin metabolic capacity, a significant elevation in production is needed. This occurs when there is marked haemolysis. Numerous causes of a haemolytic anaemia exist.
- Hepatic causes are those in which the liver's ability to handle bilirubin is impaired, either in the process of glucuronidation or the excretion into small intrahepatic bile ductules and ducts.
- Post-hepatic causes of jaundice are conditions that obstruct the extrahepatic biliary tree.

This scheme yields the conditions listed in Table 33.1.

Gilbert's syndrome is mild, quite common and tends only to manifest when the body is suffering from an intercurrent illness. It is due to reduced levels of the glucuronidation enzymes.

Question 6

Given the possible causes, what investigations could be relevant in determining the cause of jaundice?

Answer 6

A wide variety of investigations could be undertaken to evaluate the cause of jaundice. However, the history and examination should help to narrow down the differential diagnosis and permit the investigations that are requested to be focused on the likely causes in any given patient.

LIVER FUNCTION TESTS

The basic liver function tests (LFTs) are bilirubin, albumin, alanine transaminase (ALT), alkaline phosphatase (alk phos or ALP) and gamma glutamyl transferase (GGT). The last three of these are enzymes.

Two main patterns of disordered LFTs are described. In the 'hepatic' picture, the ALT and GGT are markedly raised; the ALP is normal to mildly raised. The hepatic picture occurs when the emphasis on the disease process is hepatocyte damage and is therefore accompanied by leakage of intrahepatocyte enzymes into the blood.

The 'cholestatic or biliary' pattern features a significantly raised ALP and bilirubin with a normal to mildly

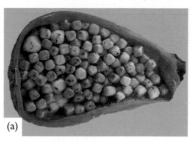 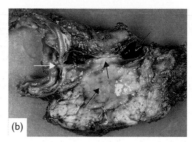

(a)   (b)

Figure 33.3 (a) Typical pale yellow mixed gallstones in gallbladder. (b) Seventy per cent of pancreatic adenocarcinomas arise in the head of the pancreas and present with obstructive jaundice due to tumour (blue arrow) compressing the lower part of the common bile duct (red arrow), as it passes through the pancreas (black arrow) and joins with the pancreatic main duct before opening into the duodenum at the ampulla of Vater (yellow arrow).

Table 33.1 Causes of jaundice	
Pre-hepatic	Haemolysis
	Drugs
Hepatic	Gilbert's syndrome
	Crigler–Najjar syndrome
	Dubin–Johnson syndrome
	Rotor syndrome
	Hepatitis
	Cirrhosis
	Drugs
	Primary biliary cirrhosis
	Biliary atresia
	Hepatic infiltration
	Sepsis
Post-hepatic	Primary sclerosing cholangitis
	Gallstones
	Biliary stricture
	Cholangiocarcinoma
	Porta hepatitis lymph nodes
	Ampullary carcinoma
	Pancreatic carcinoma
	Pancreatitis
	Drugs

elevated ALT and GGT. This combination is found when the disease process focuses on the biliary system, such as an obstructive process. The hepatocytes are not particularly damaged, so elevation of ALT and GGT is fairly mild. However, bilirubin cannot be excreted, so its levels rise. In addition, ALP is a biliary system-associated enzyme and is therefore vulnerable if the pathology is centred on this part of the system.

DETAILED BILIRUBIN

Bilirubin can be separated into its conjugated and non-conjugated components. A raised non-conjugated bilirubin implies pre-hepatic disease or defective hepatic conjugation. If the conjugated bilirubin is elevated, this suggests an obstructive element and/or damage to hepatocytes.

The presence of urobilinogen in the urine implies that at least some bilirubin is reaching the gastro-intestinal tract.

INTERNATIONAL NORMALIZED RATIO (INR)

The INR is a very useful measure of current hepatic synthetic function. A deranged INR would suggest significant impairment of hepatic synthetic function at that point in time. By contrast, the half-life of albumin makes it a poor marker of acute hepatic synthetic function.

VIRAL SEROLOGY

Jaundice is a feature of many cases of acute viral hepatitis and some cases of chronic viral hepatitis. It should be remembered that viruses other than hepatitis viruses A–E can cause hepatitis, as can other non-viral infections.

HAEMOLYSIS

Investigation of the cause of haemolytic anaemia can be complicated, but there are investigations that can be helpful in determining if haemolysis is occurring.

- The blood film may display fragmented erythrocytes.
- The reticulocyte count will be increased because the bone marrow releases reticulocytes in an attempt to maintain haemoglobin levels.
- Free haemoglobin is bound to plasma proteins known as haptoglobins. The haptoglobin–haemoglobin complex is removed by the reticuloendothelial system. Therefore, in haemolysis, haptoglobin levels are low because they are being consumed.

- The Coombs test specifically investigates for auto-antibodies against erythrocytes.

IMAGING

Hepatobiliary ultrasound, CT scans and MRI scans can help to localize obstructing mass lesions. Ultrasound is also useful for detecting gallstones and dilatation of the biliary system and has the advantages of being relatively quick to perform and not requiring ionizing radiation.

ENDOSCOPIC RETROGRADE CHOLANGIOPANCREATOGRAPHY (ERCP)

This is an image-assisted endoscopic technique in which the duodenal ampulla is cannulated and radio-opaque dye introduced into the biliary system and pancreatic duct. The endoscopic approach can also be used to retrieve gallstones from the common bile duct, place stents across strictures and increase the size of the ampullary orifice (sphincterotomy).

LIVER BIOPSY

A liver biopsy can offer precise information as to the diagnosis and stage of a disease but should generally be reserved until other investigations have greatly narrowed down the possibilities.

Question 7

Returning to this patient, he also has a history of weight loss of 5 kg over the last month, combined with a constant central upper abdominal pain that has a particularly unpleasant quality to it. On examination, in addition to the jaundice the patient has a palpable gallbladder. What is the likely diagnosis?

Answer 7

The clinical picture is strongly suggestive of pancreatic carcinoma. Courvoisier's law states that if a patient is jaundiced and the gallbladder is palpable and distended then the cause is more likely to be obstruction of the biliary system by a malignant tumour than obstruction by gallstones. The properties of the pain are typical of a pancreatic source. The weight loss is marked and in a patient of this age indicates that malignancy should be considered as the cause.

Question 8

What is the main type of pancreatic carcinoma?

Answer 8

The majority of pancreatic carcinomas are adenocarcinomas of the ductal system. Other types also exist.

Question 9

What other symptom might this patient or other patients with jaundice have?

Answer 9

The deposition of bilirubin in the skin can cause pruritus.

Question 10

What other complications can occur in chronic obstructive jaundice?

Answer 10

Bile is important in the absorption of fat and fat-soluble vitamins from the small bowel. Long-term obstructive jaundice can cause malabsorption and deficiencies of the fat-soluble vitamins (vitamins A, D, E and K).

Secondary biliary cirrhosis may develop in long-term obstructive jaundice because bile accumulates in the liver and damages it. Chronic, persisting damage to the liver is the basic process underlying most of the causes of cirrhosis.

Question 11

What complication can develop in jaundiced neonates?

Answer 11

The neonatal brain is very vulnerable to damage from unconjugated bilirubin and once levels exceed $340\,\mu mol/L$ the syndrome of kernicterus can develop due to deposition of bilirubin in the basal ganglia. The majority of affected neonates die within a couple of weeks and many of the survivors have marked psychomotor developmental retardation with extrapyramidal features and deafness.

A TUTORIAL ON GLOMERULONEPHRITIS
A Sarah McKenzie Case

The nephrology attachment took place in the fourth year of the MBBS course at Sarah's medical school. As with all of the attachments, there was an exam at the end of the firm. By the time that they sat finals, students needed to have passed each of these end of attachment exams. The exam at the end of the nephrology firm was the most notorious.

Although Sarah had been aware of the existence of the pathology museum since the first year of her course, it was only during her revision for her exams at the end of her third year that she had belatedly come to appreciate its usefulness. The pots arranged by organ system on the shelves each offered a place of entry to explore a particular topic and Sarah found the calm atmosphere of the museum conducive to study.

Sarah sat at a table by the renal specimens and took out her notes and textbooks that she hoped would guide her through the infamous waters of glomerulonephritis.

One of the histopathology consultants, Mark Southend, was inspecting the neuropathology specimens in order to select those he wished to employ in some forthcoming teaching. Ten minutes after Sarah had arrived he noticed her shaking her head over her books, as if despairing at their contents.

'Are you okay there?' asked Dr Southend.

'I'm trying to do glomerulonephritis,' replied Sarah. 'I've got my renal firm exam coming up.'

'Say no more,' smiled Dr Southend sympathetically. 'Can I help?'

Sarah was glad of the offer, but was uncertain where to begin. 'There are so many sorts and it's difficult to see how they're different and where they relate to how patients present.'

'Yes. It's a real wood for the trees situation,' sympathized Dr Southend. 'Let's get back to the basics. What's the function of the glomerulus?'

'It filters the blood to start the process of making urine.'

'Yep. What doesn't normally pass through the filter?'

'Cells and proteins.'

Table 34.1 Investigations used in renal disease

Investigation	Reason
Urea and electrolytes	
Potassium	The kidney is the main route of excretion of excess potassium ions. In acute renal failure, hyperkalaemia can develop and may reach life-threatening levels quickly. Frequent monitoring of potassium levels is therefore essential
Sodium	Most disorders of renal function have little impact on sodium levels. Close monitoring is nevertheless crucial if large volumes of fluid are given in acute renal failure secondary to fluid loss and in dialysis. Sodium levels are also vital in diabetes insipidus and the syndrome of inappropriate ADH secretion
Urea	Urea is a nitrogenous waste product of proteins that is synthesized by the liver and excreted by the kidney. It provides a measure of the severity of the renal impairment in acute and chronic renal failure
Creatinine	Creatinine is derived from muscle and normal levels exhibit racial variability. It is elevated in acute and chronic renal impairment. Note that allowance should be made in people with little muscle mass
Full blood count	
Haemoglobin	The kidney synthesizes erythropoietin, which stimulates the production of erythrocytes by the bone marrow. In chronic renal failure, erythropoietin production is reduced and anaemia can result
White cell count	The white cell count is useful if an infective or inflammatory cause is suspected for the renal dysfunction, although it is non-specific. It is also helpful as a measure of bone marrow function if primary bone marrow pathology is suspected as the cause of anaemia in a patient with renal failure
Platelets	As with the white cell count, the platelet count does not have a specific role, but is vital if a renal biopsy is contemplated, or a disorder of clotting is related to the renal dysfunction, for example hypercoaguability in nephrotic syndrome

Table 34.1 *(Continued)*

Investigation	Reason
Clotting	As for platelets
Calcium and phosphate	The kidney activates vitamin D. This activation is impaired in chronic renal failure. Hypocalcaemia then develops and is accompanied by a rise in the levels of parathyroid hormone. As a consequence, phosphate levels rise. Magnesium should also be monitored
Liver function tests	The main indication for these is to determine the albumin level. Many hospitals will include albumin levels in the 'bone profile' that measures calcium and phosphate. If the albumin level is low, it is helpful to know the other liver function tests if considering a primary liver disorder
Lipids	The nephrotic syndrome is associated with hyperlipidaemia
Arterial blood gases	The kidney is essential in the regulation of acid–base balance. A metabolic acidosis develops in acute renal failure
Urine dipstick	This is a very simple procedure that can be performed at the bedside and is often considered to be part of the examination rather than an investigation as such. The test yields qualitative rather than quantitative information, but is a good way to screen for proteinuria
Urine output	This is really a form of bedside monitoring rather than an investigation but must be mentioned due to its importance. Accurate measurement of the hourly urine output is vital in a patient who has acute renal failure. Catheterization aids this process. Urine output can given an indication of the progress of the renal failure
24-hour urine collection	The analysis of a patient's entire collected urine output from a 24-hour period is one of the more renal specific investigations. It can yield information about the degree of proteinuria and is part of the measurement of renal function through the creatinine clearance. It also has uses outside nephrology in endocrinology, such as the assessment of urinary catecholamines in phaeochromocytoma
Autoantibodies	These are discussed in Case 38, A chronic autoimmune disease (p. 147). Those of most relevance to nephrology are ANCA (antineutrophil cytoplasmic antibodies) in vasculitis and ANA (antinuclear antibodies, particularly those to double-stranded DNA) for systemic lupus erythematosus
Complement	Complement levels may be altered in systemic lupus erythematosus
Immunoglobulins and serum electrophoresis	Like complement levels, this is another focused test, this time one that is called upon if myeloma is suspected as the cause of the renal impairment
Imaging	Diverse imaging modalities may be required. A plain abdominal X-ray is helpful if ureteric calculi are suspected. Ultrasound is useful in evaluation of obstruction and hydronephrosis, as well as contributing to the evaluation of tumours. Nuclear medicine scans can provide data regarding the proportion of the overall renal excretory function that is contributed by each of the kidneys. This is important if nephrectomy is contemplated
Renal biopsy	Histopathological examination is important in a variety of renal conditions, particularly the investigation of nephrotic syndrome/glomerulonephritis and in assessing transplant rejection. Renal biopsies are one of the few areas in histopathology where electron microscopy retains a role. Comprehensive clinical details to accompany the specimen are essential
Others	The causes of renal dysfunction can be diverse and some of these will have specific investigations that are unique to them, so the above list is not exhaustive. However, the above investigations should allow establishment of the basic parameters relating to the renal impairment and help to guide any further specific tests

It is important to remember that whenever a test is requested, there is reasoning behind the selection of that test. The information provided by the investigation must be relevant to the patient's condition(s) and have the potential to alter the management of that patient. This concept applies both to giving answers in an examination and when dealing with patients.

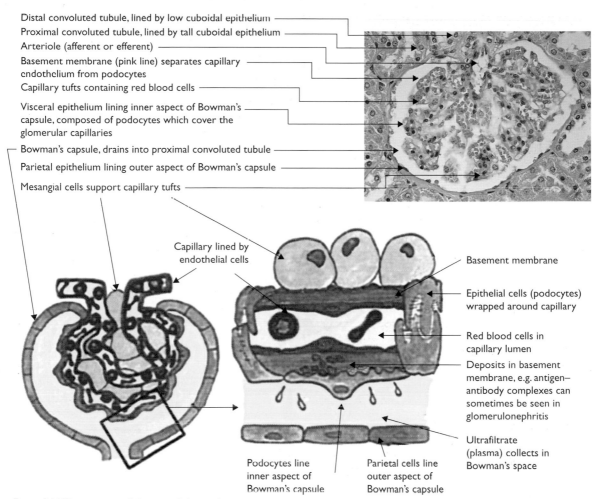

Distal convoluted tubule, lined by low cuboidal epithelium
Proximal convoluted tubule, lined by tall cuboidal epithelium
Arteriole (afferent or efferent)
Basement membrane (pink line) separates capillary endothelium from podocytes
Capillary tufts containing red blood cells
Visceral epithelium lining inner aspect of Bowman's capsule, composed of podocytes which cover the glomerular capillaries
Bowman's capsule, drains into proximal convoluted tubule
Parietal epithelium lining outer aspect of Bowman's capsule
Mesangial cells support capillary tufts

Capillary lined by endothelial cells

Basement membrane

Epithelial cells (podocytes) wrapped around capillary

Red blood cells in capillary lumen

Deposits in basement membrane, e.g. antigen–antibody complexes can sometimes be seen in glomerulonephritis

Ultrafiltrate (plasma) collects in Bowman's space

Podocytes line inner aspect of Bowman's capsule

Parietal cells line outer aspect of Bowman's capsule

Figure 34.1 The structure of the normal glomerulus.

'Yes, cells and large molecules, which are mainly proteins. In particular, the glomerulus shouldn't let albumin through. What parts are there to the glomerulus? There aren't that many.'

Sarah had not considered the glomerulus from this perspective before. 'Well, it sits in the Bowman's capsule and there must be blood vessels in it to provide the blood that gets filtered.'

'That's a start. Are the blood vessels just floating around in the breeze of the filtrate, or do they have any support?'

'There must be some sort of stroma,' answered Sarah. The mire of terms of nephrology swirled in her mind and one struggled to the surface. 'Is that the mesangium?'

'Yes. The mesangial cells hold it all together. What about the filtration? What keeps the proteins back but lets fluid and small molecules through?'

'That's the podocytes with their foot processes.'

Dr Southend nodded. 'They sit on the outside of the capillaries. Their foot processes have a negative charge which helps to repel proteins. That's it, really. You have the capillaries, the mesangium and the podocytes forming the glomerular capillary tuft sat in the Bowman's capsule. The Bowman's capsule has an outer layer of parietal pleura and the cells in that, plus the mesangium are the only ones in the system that can divide to any real degree. The other key player is the basement membrane between the capillaries and podocytes.'

'And that's it?'

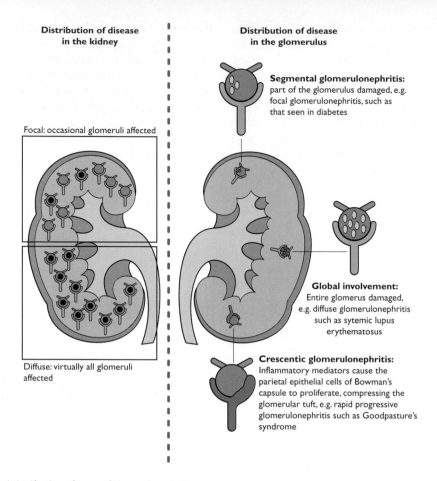

Figure 34.2 Broad classification of types of glomerulonephritis.

'For the glomerulus, yes. So how do those five components get transformed into a subject that drives medical students up the wall?'

Sarah smiled at the empathetic joke. 'That's my problem.'

'Okay, have you noticed any similarities between the diseases you've been reading about?'

'Not in terms of a cause. There's this stuff about immune complexes and antibodies, but they're all diverse.'

'In some senses yes, but in others not so. You're right that there are many different patterns and secondary causes, but there are common themes. Basically, there's an inflammatory response directed against the glomerulus. Antigens, antibodies and immune complexes are at the heart of it.

'In some sorts of glomerulonephritis, the immune complexes are generated outside the glomerulus but become trapped in it and excite an inflammatory response there. As soon as you mention immune complexes, you're almost automatically implicating complement in the equation. You can see this aetiology in things like Henoch–Schonlein purpura and SLE nephritis. Other times, such as in Goodpasture's disease, only autoantibodies are formed outside the glomerulus but these target the glomerulus. When they reach the glomerulus you get the predictable inflammatory response that you'd expect when lots of antibodies hit their target antigen. In Goodpasture's disease, the antibodies are directed against the glomerular basement membrane.

'Lots of the primary glomerulonephritises operate in these ways and so do many of the secondary ones, but you also have to remember to include specific diseases of blood vessels, like vasculitis and thrombotic thrombocytopenic purpura, in which you have a small vessel-mediated disease process, again often autoimmune.'

'That's where Wegener's granulomatosis comes in,' observed Sarah.

'Yes. So you've got a glomerulus that's under inflammatory attack from antibodies, or immune complexes, or because something's harming its capillaries. Where in the glomerulus the immune complexes impact, or where the antibodies are targeted, determines whether the glomerulus responds by producing more mesangium or duplicating or thickening its basement membrane around the immune complexes and those changes from the basis of the names like membranous, membranoproliferative and mesangial.'

'Where does crescentic glomerulonephritis fit in, please?' inquired Sarah. 'People talk about it and say that it's serious but it crops up all over the place.'

'Crescentic glomerulonephritis is just a descriptive term. Anything that causes glomerulonephritis can cause crescents. Crescents are the parietal pleural cells proliferating in response to the glomerular injury. It's important because the crescents compress the glomerular capillary tuft and damage it and can destroy it quickly. Different causes of glomerulonephritis have different propensities to cause crescents. Ones like Goodpasture's and Wegener's are among the more likely and can wreck kidneys very quickly, so if a patient has crescents, you need to act rapidly and typically aggressively. But that's what they are, a particular response to injury that indicates a serious threat to renal function. The next thing to discuss is how these pathological processes disrupt renal function and in what ways.' Dr Southend paused to consider how to move onto this new topic. 'Okay, how do you think the podocytes feel about all this nonsense breaking out in the glomerulus?'

'They're not going to be too happy,' replied Sarah, following Dr Southend's colloquial lead.

'Exactly. They tend to get cheesed off and can't do their job properly. In one sort of glomerulonephritis, minimal change disease, there's virtually nothing to see, hence the name, but the podocytes don't work properly. If you look with electron microscopy, their foot processes might be a little further apart than they should and it's said that they lose their negative charge. Now, if the podocytes don't work properly and their job is to regulate what can and can't be filtered, what do you think happens?'

'The glomerulus leaks.'

'Yes. Add in direct damage to capillaries and the mesangium in more aggressive diseases and you can see that things can really get leaky. So what leaks out?'

Nephrotic syndrome ('O'):
- Proteinuria >3.5 g/day
- Oedema (due to hypoalbuminaemia) – especially marked around eyes
- Hyperlipidaemia – the liver synthesizes extra liporoteins as a non-specific response to decreased plasma oncotic pressure (due to proteinuria), especially LDL.

Risk associated with nephrotic syndrome:
- Hypercoaguability of the blood, with thrombosis of renal or deep veins.
- Atherosclerosis (high LDL and cholesterol levels)
- Infection (loss of antibodies in the gamma globulin fraction of plasma)

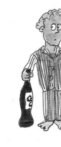

Nephritic syndrome ('I')
- Haematuria – can give urine a 'smoky' or 'cola' colour
- Oliguria
- Hypertension
- Less than 2g proteinurea per day
- Slight oedema

Figure 34.3 The salient features of nephritic and nephrotic syndrome.

'Proteins and blood.'

'Which brings us onto the nephrotic and nephritic syndromes. You can probably guess the next question.'

'What's the difference?'

'Right.'

'Nephrotic syndrome occurs when you lose protein,' Sarah paused to recall the precise number, 'At least 3.5 g per day. In nephritic you have haematuria and hypertension but don't lose much protein.'

'Basically. People dispute the precise figure for the amount of protein loss, but most settle around 3.5 g. Others take a more pragmatic approach and say that the protein loss is of a sufficient level to cause oedema. Which disease is nephritic syndrome mainly associated with?'

'That's, erm, post-streptococcal glomerulonephritis,' stated Sarah.

'Yes, it's the weird cross-reactivity thing. If you want to look really smart and give the subtypes of streptococcus, just give the square numbers up to 49, but miss out 9, 16 and 36.'

Sarah nodded, aware that examiners would be impressed by this trivia.

'Somebody was probably having a laugh with the terminology,' resumed Dr Southend. 'Nephrotic and nephritic look like they're designed to cause confusion, but you can simplify it down to most types of glomerulonephritis giving nephrotic syndrome and in any case, the patient's presentation defines whether its nephrotic or nephritic, not the type of glomerulonephritis. I suppose if you want to remember it, nephrotic syndrome gives you oedema which starts with an o and makes you swell up like an o and o is in nephrotic but not nephritic. I've already given the game away with oedema in nephrotic syndrome but what else happens?'

'You can get pleural effusions and ascites,' replied Sarah, continuing with the theme of a reduced plasma protein pressure.

'Good. What else? What might the liver do to try to cope with the loss of proteins?'

'I'm not sure.'

'Don't worry. It pumps out lipoproteins to try to hold things together, so the patient gets hyperlipidaemia. There's also a procoagulant tendency, possibly because you tend to get that in inflammation generally, combined with the liver throwing fibrinogen into the fray to try to keep the oncotic pressure up, as well as a loss of anticoagulant proteins through the damaged glomeruli. Albumin can oppose platelet aggregation and the kidney is losing albumin at a rate of knots. All of this means that the frequency of venous thrombosis, including renal vein thrombosis can really be very significant.'

'Can I ask about the terms diffuse and focal and segmental, please?'

'Sure. Diffuse means that all glomeruli are affected, focal means that only some are and segmental indicates that within an affected glomerulus, only part of it is involved. Did you have a particular disease in mind?'

'Focal segmental glomerulonephritis was one I'd heard about.'

'What had you heard?'

'That you get nephrotic syndrome and it comes back in transplants.'

'That's the key concept and is probably the place to finish before I overload you. Although the classification is often confusing, the importance of the different types of glomerulonephritis is that they have different prognoses, different rates of progression and different recurrence rates in transplants. The different secondary causes of glomerulonephritis tend to favour certain patterns of glomerulonephritis, although ultimately you need to keep an open mind and investigate widely to make sure that there isn't an underlying cause that is actually eminently treatable before the kidney is permanently wrecked. I think I'd better leave it there. That's kind of an overview for you and you can use it to hang the details on.'

PART 4

TREATMENT

A 65-year-old man presents to his GP with a four-month history of tiredness and a sensation of fullness in the left side of his abdomen. Examination is unremarkable other than splenomegaly which extends towards the right iliac fossa.

Question 1

What are the causes of massive splenomegaly?

Answer 1

This is a popular exam question as there are only a handful of typical causes of massive splenomegaly:

- myelofibrosis
- chronic myeloid leukaemia
- leishmaniasis
- chronic malaria
- gaucher's disease.

Assorted other causes of lesser degrees of splenomegaly exist, but tend not to produce a massive degree of enlargement.

Question 2

The GP requests a full blood count (see Investigations box below). Which of the diagnoses is/are most likely?

Investigations

Hb	10.9 g/dL
WCC	65×10^9/L (neutrophils 59×10^9/L)
Platelets	173×10^9/L
MCV	84 fL
MHC	30.8 pg
MCHC	33.1 g/dL

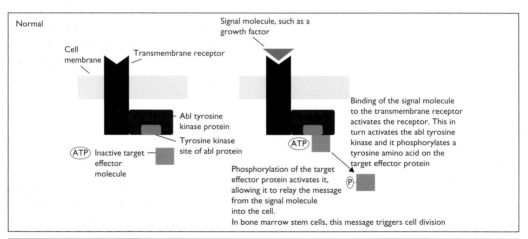

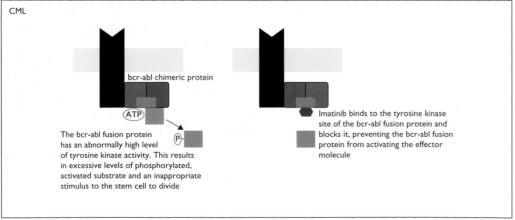

Figure 35.1 The action of imatinib, a 'designer drug' which was specifically manufactured to block a tyrosine kinase receptor expressed in chronic myeloid leukaemia. The same receptor has since been found to be expressed in other tumours, which are also responsive to this drug (see Table 35.1).

Answer 2

The markedly elevated white cell count (WCC) makes chronic myeloid leukaemia the most likely diagnosis of the five causes of massive splenomegaly. The early stages of myelofibrosis can also be associated with leukocytosis, although not usually of this degree.

Question 3

The patient is referred to a haematologist and a bone marrow trephine is performed. The trephine is hypercellular and shows trilinear haematopoiesis with abundant representatives of all three cell lineages, although myelopoietic elements dominate. The Philadelphia chromosome is detected. What is the diagnosis?

Answer 3

Chronic myeloid leukaemia (CML).

Note that the presence or absence of the Philadelphia chromosome is a key diagnostic criterion in the myeloproliferative disorders.

Question 4

What is the Philadelphia chromosome?

Answer 4

The Philadelphia chromosome is an abnormal form of chromosome 22 that is the result of a translocation between the long arm of chromosome 9 and the long arm of chromosome 22. This translocation fuses the coding region for the *abl* gene of chromosome 9 with the *bcr* region of chromosome 22.

Question 5

The *abl* gene codes a tyrosine kinase. What alterations in function could happen to a tyrosine kinase protein as the result of a mutation (either a translocation or other type of mutation)?

Answer 5

Mutation of a tyrosine kinase could result in a complete loss of function, reduced function or overactivity.

Question 6

What is the basic role of tyrosine kinases?

Answer 6

Tyrosine kinases form part of a variety of cell surface receptor systems. Binding of the appropriate ligand to the receptor activates the tyrosine kinase, resulting in phosphorylation of a target protein which in turn relays a signal to the cell. In some tyrosine kinase receptor systems, this signal is one that contributes to the regulation of cell division.

Question 7

The *bcr-abl* fusion gene encodes a tyrosine kinase that has a much greater activity than normal. How could this explain the myeloproliferative process of CML?

Answer 7

CML is a clonal myeloproliferative bone marrow stem cell disorder in which there is an increase in the number of neutrophils and their precursors in the bone marrow and peripheral blood (the stem cell also generates cells of the erythroid and megakaryocyte series). If a bone marrow stem cell acquires the Philadelphia chromosome, the greatly enhanced tyrosine kinase activity of the *bcr-abl* fusion protein provides an excessive drive to the cell to divide. However, at this stage, there is no blockage to the maturation pathways of the daughter cells, so CML features an excess of mature forms (compared with acute myeloid leukaemia (AML) and acute lymphoblastic leukaemia (ALL) in which significant maturation is not encountered).

Question 8

What possible avenue of treatment does the role of the *bcr-abl* fusion gene tyrosine kinase suggest?

Answer 8

In view of the central role of the abnormal tyrosine kinase in CML, therapy that targeted this abnormal tyrosine kinase could block the disregulated cell division and control the disease. Until relatively recently, this specific treatment was not available, but there is now available a monoclonal antibody (imatinib, trade name Glivec) which is directed against the abnormal tyrosine kinase and neutralizes its actions. Imatinib is highly effective in returning the blood count to normal and can render the bone marrow negative for the Philadelphia chromosome (the mutated stem cells no longer have a growth advantage over normal stem cells).

Some other examples of targeted cancer therapies are listed in Table 35.1.

Question 9

Under what circumstances may the effectiveness of imatinib become impaired?

Table 35.1 Examples of targeted cancer therapies

Agent	Target	Process targeted	Cancer type
Monoclonal antibodies			
Bevacizumab (Avastin)	Vascular endotheial growth factor	Angiogenesis	Colorectal (metastatic)
Cetuximab (Erbitux)	Epidermal growth factor receptor	Growth factor signalling	Colorectal
Trastuzumab (Herceptin)[a]	HER2 receptor	Growth factor signalling	Breast
Rituximab (Mabthera)	CD20 receptor	Induces cell death	B cell lymphoma
Small molecule inhibitors			
Imatinib (Glivec)[b]	Bcl-Abl fusion protein; Kit	Growth factor signalling	Chronic myeloid leukaemia; gastrointestinal stromal tumours
Erlotinib (Tarceva)	Epidermal growth factor receptor	Growth factor signalling	Non-small cell lung cancer
Bortezomib (Velcade)	Proteosome	Multiple processes affected	Multiple myeloma

[a]The monoclonal antibody therapy Herceptin (trastuzumab) targets the cell surface HER2 growth factor receptor (also known as c-ErbB2). HER2 is overexpressed in around a quarter of all breast cancers. Herceptin has been recommended for treating metastatic breast cancer for some time, in combination with chemotherapy.

[b]Glivec (imatinib mesylate) is a tyrosine kinase inhibitor that prevents activation of the Bcr-Abl protein, and, as a result, inhibits cell proliferation and promotes apoptosis. In England and Wales it is now recommended as the first-line treatment for adults with chronic phase BCR-ABL-positive CML and chemoresistant gastrointestinal stromal tumours, where it targets the Kit receptor.

Adapted from CRC UK, Genes and Cancer. http://info.cancerresearchuk.org/cancerstats/causes/genes/diagnosisandtreatment/?a=5441

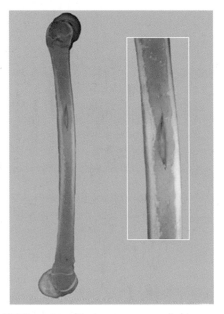

Figure 35.2 Expansion of the bone marrow cavity by a homogeneous leukaemic infiltrate, seen at higher magnification (inset). In an adult, only the shaft of the femur contains red bone marrow. Here there is featureless fleshy tumour replacing and expanding the marrow cavity, including the femoral head and neck.

Answer 9

CML has the ability to transform to an acute leukaemia, either myeloblastic (70–80 per cent) or lymphoblastic (20–30 per cent) and this is a common cause of death in CML. The additional mutations accumulated by the acute leukaemic cells negate some or all of their dependence on the drive provided by the *bcr-abl* product. Therefore, while imatinib may still be employed, the appropriate chemotherapy for ALL or AML must be added. Even then, the prognosis of transformed CML remains poor and is typically worse than that for primary ALL or AML.

Question 10

Why could a patient with CML require allopurinol?

Answer 10

Allopurinol is employed in the treatment of gout. Patients with CML have a significant increase in the turnover of nucleic acids and this results in elevated levels of uric acid. In some patients, this will precipitate gout.

A 23-year-old woman presents to her GP with a four-week history of increasing lethargy and easy bruising. She has also remarked that her last period, which was two weeks ago, was unusually heavy. On examination, the woman is pale and has scattered bruises. There are no focal abnormalities in the cardiovascular, respiratory, abdominal or neurological systems. The GP requests some initial blood tests. The laboratory at the local hospital telephones these through shortly after they are confirmed, as well as faxing a printed copy of the finalized report.

Investigations

Hb	5.2 g/dL
WCC	1.3×10^9/L
Neutrophils	0.3×10^9/L
Platelets	15×10^9/L
MCV	107 fL
MCH	30.1 pg
MCHC	33.5 g/dL
INR	1.1
APTTR	1.0

Question 1

What abnormalities are present?

Answer 1

The patient has pancytopenia. This term indicates the combination of anaemia, leukopenia and thrombocytopenia.

Additional details in this case are the neutropenia and a macrocytic anaemia.

Question 2

Where are erythrocytes, granulocytes and platelets produced?

Answer 2

In the bone marrow. The bone marrow synthesizes these three cellular elements of the peripheral blood. This is referred to as trilineage haematopoiesis and comprises erythropoiesis (red cells), myelopoiesis (granulocytes) and megakaryopoiesis (platelets via megakaryocytes).

Question 3

What conditions could cause the bone marrow to fail?

Answer 3

The causes of bone marrow failure can be divided into the categories of a loss of the normal contents of the bone marrow, replacement of the bone marrow by other tissue or dysfunction of the bone marrow:

- Loss of normal contents
  - aplastic anaemia
- Replacement by other tissue
  - haematological malignancy (leukaemia, myeloma, sometimes lymphoma)
  - secondary tumour, usually a carcinoma
  - myelofibrosis (replacement by fibrous tissue)

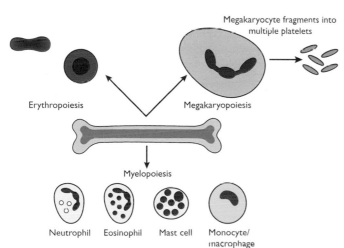

Figure 36.1 Summary of the normal pathways involved in haematopoiesis, which is the generation of blood cells by the bone marrow. The bone marrow stem cell gives rise to specialized myeloid, lymphoid and erythroid precursor cells, which differentiate to form mature cells under the influence of colony-stimulating factors and local factors, such as cytokines or erythropoietin. The bone marrow stromal cells can secrete local hormones and therefore are not the simple 'packing material' they were once considered to be. Platelets are formed from megakaryocyte cytoplasm and have no nuclear material. Erythrocytes normally lose their nuclear material prior to entering the blood.

- amyloidosis
- Gaucher's disease
• Ineffective haematopoiesis
  - myelodysplasia
  - megaloblastic anaemia
  - inherited disorders.

Question 4

What other disorders could cause pancytopenia?

Answer 4

Even if the bone marrow is working normally, cytopenias in the peripheral blood can result from either destruction of the blood cells after they are synthesized or their pooling (sequestration) somewhere.

• Peripheral destruction of blood cells
  - autoimmune
  - paroxysmal nocturnal haemoglobinuria
• Peripheral sequestration
  - hypersplenism.

Question 5

The GP contacts the patient and the local haematology team and arranges urgent admission that day for investigation and treatment of the patient's pancytopenia. Assorted investigations are undertaken, but the key procedure in this patient's case is a bone marrow trephine and aspirate. Figure 36.2 shows a normal trephine and one that could have come from this patient. What is the striking difference?

Answer 5

The patient's trephine is effectively devoid of haematopoietic cells and does not show replacement by an abnormal infiltrate.

Question 6

A diagnosis of aplastic anaemia is made. What is this condition and what are its causes?

Answer 6

Aplastic anaemia is a disease in which there is a chronic pancytopenia due to hypoplasia of the haematopoietic bone marrow. There are assorted causes:

• Congenital – various disorders, including Fanconi anaemia
• Idiopathic
• Viral
• Drugs – e.g. gold, chloramphenicol (mainly historical)
• Chemotherapy
• Toxic chemicals – e.g. benzene
• Radiation
• Associated with haematological malignancy
• Associated with paroxysmal nocturnal haemoglobinuria.

Question 7

What complications does this woman face?

Answer 7

The patient has severe anaemia with the consequent problems of impaired oxygen carriage and delivery, cardiovascular strain due to a hyperdynamic circulation and marked vulnerability to any further haemoglobin loss.

The patient's menorrhagia and easy bruising means that her thrombocytopenia is demonstrably of a sufficient degree to compromise blood clotting. This bleeding tendency could exacerbate the anaemia. There is also a danger of a spontaneous intracranial haemorrhage.

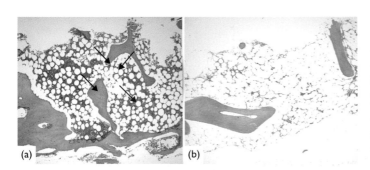

(a)   (b)

Figure 36.2 (a) Normal bone marrow. The bone trabeculae (black arrows) enclose marrow spaces in which haematopoietic tissue (red arrow) and mature adipose tissue (blue arrow) are present. The proportion occupied by the haematopoietic tissue decreases with age. (b) Bone marrow in aplastic anaemia. The bone marrow is formed almost entirely of mature adipose tissue. Haematopoietic elements are inconspicuous.

The leukopenia renders the patient susceptible to infection. The neutropenia in particular makes the patient vulnerable to bacterial infection and fungal infection, especially of the opportunistic type.

It should also be remembered that if there is an underlying cause for the aplastic anaemia, this could have other specific complications beyond that of bone marrow failure.

Question 8

What issues should treatment address?

Answer 8

There are two main arms to the treatment of aplastic anaemia. The bone marrow failure means that replacement of the missing cellular components of the blood is required. In parallel to this is the aim to restore normal haematopoiesis.

Question 9

How can this be achieved?

Answer 9a

Of the three elements of the pancytopenia, the anaemia is the easiest to address. Blood transfusions can be given as necessary and the donated red cells have a reasonable half-life within the recipient. Problems can arise after multiple transfusions because the recipient can develop numerous antibodies to minor blood group antigens, making cross-matching and locating units of blood harder.

Platelet transfusion can be employed to correct the thrombocytopenia, but infused platelets have a

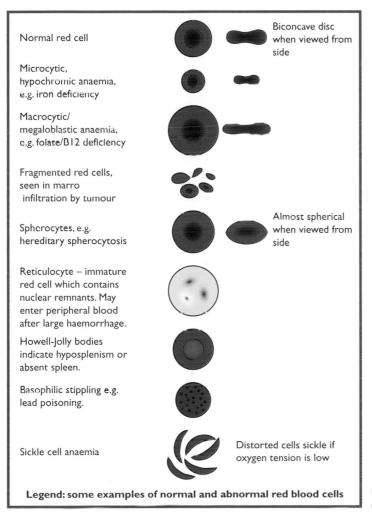

Legend: some examples of normal and abnormal red blood cells

Figure 36.3 Red blood cell appearances in different types of anaemia.

disappointing half-life within the patient (perhaps only a few days). Platelet transfusion tends to be reserved for thrombocytopenic patients who have significant bleeding. However, if levels are very low, transfusion may be also given prophylactically.

Replacing leukocytes is the most difficult. Leukocyte (buffy coat) infusion is ineffective and seldom employed. Thus, unlike red cells and platelets, direct replacement by transfusion is not an option. Instead, attempts can be made to stimulate the patient's own myelopoiesis with injections of growth factors such as G-CSF (granulocyte colony-stimulating factor) but this can be of limited efficacy. The risk of opportunistic infection becomes especially marked when the neutrophil count falls below $0.5 \times 10^9/L$.

While it may not be possible to replace/regenerate the neutrophils effectively, the dangers of opportunistic infection can be reduced by controlling the patient's environment. This involves the use of special side rooms and reverse barrier nursing in order to minimize the chances of the patient encountering a pathogen.

If a patient with neutropenia does become febrile, or develop an infection, prompt and aggressive antimicrobial treatment is essential because the patient's depleted immune response means that the infection can become overwhelming and fatal within hours.

Answer 9b

Supportive therapy cannot be continued indefinitely and it is necessary to endeavour to restore normal haematopoietic bone marrow function. This can be achieved in several ways.

If an underlying cause for the aplastic anaemia is known, this should be addressed, for example, withdrawing a causative drug.

In many cases of aplastic anaemia, the destruction of the haematopoietic cells is mediated by the patient's own immune system, specifically the lymphocyte component. Therefore, despite the existence of the neutropenia, inducing immunosuppression is often beneficial. This is in the form of antilymphocyte globulin (ALG) or antithymocyte globulin (ATG) in order to target the lymphocytes specifically.

Androgens (anabolic steroids) have been found to be helpful in some cases.

As mentioned above, growth factors such as G-CSF tend to provide supportive treatment rather than restorative.

If the above treatments fail and the aplastic anaemia is severe, bone marrow transplantation can be attempted. This requires an HLA (human leukocyte antigen)-matched donor. First-degree relatives tend to be the first place to look for a match.

Question 10

What is the prognosis?

Answer 10

The course of aplastic anaemia can be variable. Some people make an excellent recovery. However, others have a more complex course and it must be remembered that aplastic anaemia is a serious disease that can readily kill.

A PROPHYLACTIC RESECTION

Arthur McTaggart, a 46-year-old businessman, presents to his family doctor complaining of feeling exhausted. He becomes breathless on the slightest exertion and stops twice as he climbs the stairs to his second-floor office. The doctor notices that his mucous membranes are extremely pale and suspects that he is anaemic. On general systems enquiries, Arthur admits that he has begun to pass more wind than usual and that he has recently noted slime when he opens his bowels. He has never been aware of fresh blood per rectum or dark, tarry stools. He has not lost weight. There are no other symptoms of note.

On digital rectal examination, the doctor notes that the rectal mucosa feels generally lumpy, but that there is no single discrete mass.

A full blood count confirms that Arthur has a microcytic, hypochromic anaemia, most likely to be due to chronic iron loss from bleeding. In view of his gut-related symptoms the doctor refers him to the rapid access gastrointestinal clinic at the local hospital.

Mr Southern, the consultant surgeon, is astonished when on sigmoidoscopy he sees a carpet of polyps of varying size. A colonoscopy is organized for a few days' time. This confirms that the entire colon is involved by polyposis and that there is a fungating, ulcerated cancer in the caecum, confirmed by biopsy and histological examination.

Question 1

What is the link between colonic polyps and cancer?

Answer 1

The most common colonic polyps are adenomas and hyperplastic polyps. Adenomas are dysplastic, i.e. the epithelial cells show cytological and architectural characteristics similar to those seen in malignant cells, such as a high nuclear:cytoplasmic ratio, disorganized growth and increased numbers of mitoses.

Adenocarcinoma often develops within a large polyp, usually those larger than 2 cm diameter, with a villous growth pattern and high-grade dysplasia.

Hyperplastic polyps do not show dysplasia and are not regarded as pre-malignant.

After staging by CT scan, which shows no metastatic spread, Arthur undergoes a total colectomy. The histology report reads as follows:

> *Arthur McTaggart, age 46 years, Consultant Mr Southern*
> *Operation: Panproctocolectomy for familial polyposis coli*
> *with caecal adenocarcinoma.*

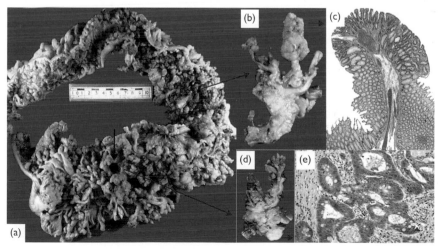

Figure 37.1 (a) Total colectomy specimen. The colon is carpeted by adenomatous polyps – tubular, tubulovillous and villous in shape – and there is an ulcerated adenocarcinoma towards the caecum (blue arrow). (b) Inset shows a slice through a polypoid region, which shows (c) the typical microscopical appearance of a tubular adenoma with low grade dysplasia. This area appears blue (because the cells show disordered maturation and have crowded nuclei). (d) Inset shows a slice taken adjacent to the ulcerated cancer in the caecum. The node and fatty tissue (red arrows) have a white appearance due to tumour infiltration. (e) Microscopy of this area shows irregular, atypical glands in the node – this is adenocarcinoma.

The 36 mm diameter ulcerated tumour identified in the caecum is a poorly differentiated adenocarcinoma which has spread to 5/42 pericolic lymph nodes and is present in a medium-sized blood vessel in the serosal fat. The apical lymph node is not involved. The retroperitoneal, peritoneal and surgical longitudinal margins are clear. The tumour has penetrated the serosa and is exposed on the peritoneal surface.

TNM stage pT4, N2 MX; Dukes' stage C1.

The remainder of the colon and rectum bear innumerable adenomatous polyps between 3 and 16 mm in diameter. Two of the larger polyps in the rectum show high-grade dysplasia and the remainder show low grade dysplasia. Intervening mucosa shows the presence of unicryptal adenomas, characteristic of familial polyposis coli.

Question 2

Mr Southern explains to Arthur the prognostic implications of these findings – what are they?

Answer 2

The TNM staging system (T = tumour, N = nodes, M = metastasis) is used throughout the body, though each site has a specific set of parameters. T4 is the most advanced degree of spread through the wall, involving breach of the peritoneal covering which means that tumour cells are liable to seed across the peritoneal cavity. More than three lymph nodes are involved, pushing this into the unwelcome N2 stage. No biopsies of putative metastases have been taken, so this is MX.

The presence of vascular invasion means that there is a risk that tumour will have spread to the liver via the portal vein, which drains the entire bowel except the anus.

This is a Dukes' stage C2 adenocarcinoma of colon, which is poorly differentiated (grade 3). Between 40–60 per cent of patients with this Dukes' stage will be alive in five years; his poor TNM parameters place him at the 40 per cent end of the survival statistics.

Mr Southern questions Arthur about his family. His mother died of bowel cancer when he was a child. Although he is estranged from his sister and two brothers, an aunt contacted them when she heard of Arthur's cancer. His sister turns out to have had a malignant polyp removed from her colon last year.

Arthur's blood is subjected to genetic analysis. This shows a germline DNA mutation in the *APC* gene.

Arthur is divorced and has not seen his only child, Jake, since he was 11 years old.

Jake, now aged 24, is contacted and invited for a consultation, at which he is advised to have a colonoscopy. This shows two small adenomatous polyps in his transverse and sigmoid colon. To his amazement, Mr Southern recommends that he undergo a total colectomy. As with his father, an ileal pouch would form a neo-rectum connected to his anus.

Question 3

Jake asks Mr Southern why he should have such radical surgery. After all, he only has two small polyps and his father had hundreds.

Answer 3

Once one adenomatous polyp has grown in a patient with familial adenomatous polyposis, the risk of a colorectal cancer supervening in at least one, if not more, of the many polyps which will soon follow is almost 100 per cent. The onset of polyps, usually in the late teenage years, is an indication for a prophylactic panproctocolectomy.

Question 4

'Why should one mutation have so much influence?' enquires Jake.

Answer 4

The *APC* gene on chromosome 5 encodes a large protein with several domains, including that for beta-catenin. Familial polyposis patients inherit a 'germline mutation' which means that all cells in the body carry one abnormal copy of the *APC* gene. However *APC* gene mutations are some of the most common and earliest found in

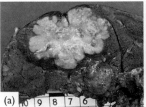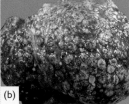

(a)   (b)

Figure 37.2 Blood-borne spread from colorectal cancer is usually first seen in the liver. (a) A solitary metastasis such as that shown here may be treatable by wedge resection, giving months to years of symptom-free remission. (b) Multiple liver metastases are non-resectable but may respond to chemotherapy for months/years.

sporadic colorectal adenocarcinomas, which are not inherited, but develop during life ('somatic mutation') – in this case only the tumour cells show the mutation and the rest of the cells in the body are normal.

One reason for the important role of the *APC* gene in colon cancer development is that, among other roles, beta-catenin affects the mitotic spindle and can alter the ability of the cell to divide its number of chromosomes equally at cell division. The risk of further mutations is therefore increased, as subsequent progeny inherit excess or deficient chromosomal segments.

Cancer is caused by a series of DNA mutations, each conferring on a cell line a growth or survival advantage, or a means of breaking away from the original tissue and spreading to distant sites. In a seminal paper in 1980, Vogelstein investigated mutations in a range of tumour suppressor genes and oncogenes and recognized a typical sequence of mutations in the adenoma–carcinoma sequence.

An alternative pathway, due to mutation in DNA mismatch repair (MMR) enzyme genes, has been described. The MMR enzymes repair DNA replicative errors prior to the completion of mitosis. They are encoded by tumour suppressor genes so both copies must be inactivated before the effects are felt. The common methods of inactivation are methylation of CpG islands or deletion of large parts of the gene during defective cell division.

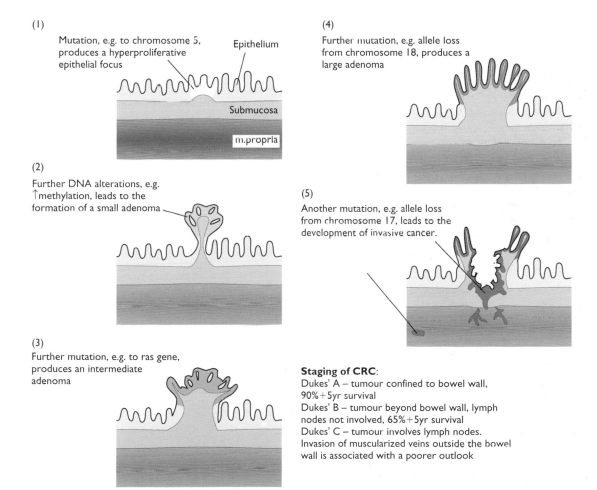

(1) Mutation, e.g. to chromosome 5, produces a hyperproliferative epithelial focus

Epithelium

Submucosa

m.propria

(2) Further DNA alterations, e.g. ↑methylation, leads to the formation of a small adenoma

(3) Further mutation, e.g. to ras gene, produces an intermediate adenoma

(4) Further mutation, e.g. allele loss from chromosome 18, produces a large adenoma

(5) Another mutation, e.g. allele loss from chromosome 17, leads to the development of invasive cancer.

Staging of CRC:
Dukes' A – tumour confined to bowel wall, 90%+5yr survival
Dukes' B – tumour beyond bowel wall, lymph nodes not involved, 65%+5yr survival
Dukes' C – tumour involves lymph nodes. Invasion of muscularized veins outside the bowel wall is associated with a poorer outlook

Figure 37.3 Traditionally accepted sequence of events involved in about 70% of colorectal cancers and in familial adenomatous polyposis (FAP). Staging utilizes the TNM and Dukes' systems. The TNM staging is described in the text.

Question 5

Jake asks if there are any other inherited cancer syndromes.

Answer 5

Inherited cancer syndromes include:

- Xeroderma pigmentosum: a rare syndrome caused by mutations in nuclear excision and repair genes. Patients with ultraviolet light-induced DNA damage cannot replace the faulty segment and develop multiple skin cancers, often in childhood.
- Li-Fraumeni syndrome: a predisposition to develop multiple primary cancers, including of the colon. Fifty per cent carry mutated p53, a tumour suppressor gene.
- *BRCA1*: this was the first of the familial breast cancer genes to be identified. Patients inherit a predisposition to develop breast, ovarian, prostate and colorectal cancers. It is a tumour suppressor gene, involved in repairing defects in other genes.
- Hereditary non-polyposis colorectal cancer (HNPCC) and familial adenomatous polyposis (FAP) as above – both rare causes of colorectal cancer (CRC).

Question 6

'If colorectal cancer is common, but familial cancer is rare, what else is thought to be important in colorectal cancer development?' asks Jake. 'And can anything prevent it?'

Answer 6

- Environmental and dietary agents including nitrosamines, fibre, stool transit time, smoking (i.e. reactive oxygen species), burned meats and smoked foods have all been implicated in CRC.
- Chronic inflammatory bowel disease: ulcerative colitis and Crohn's disease, involving frequent cycles of gut epithelial damage and repair, increase the likelihood of spontaneous mutation. Once cell division has occurred, mutations are incorporated in the genetic blueprint for the new cell and are replicated when it divides.
- Previous sporadic polyps, especially if multiple, indicate that a patient is likely to have more adenomas and may develop an adenocarcinoma. Lifelong surveillance is recommended.
- A family history of colonic cancer increases the risk in first-degree relatives. Rectal cancer is less likely to be familial. Both genetic and epigenetic factors are probably involved.
- Antioxidants such as low-dose aspirin are protective.
- A high-fibre diet is protective, probably by reducing stool transit time and thus decreasing bowel exposure to carcinogens.

Jake has the colectomy. He and his father convalesce together and become close again. Sadly, Arthur develops metastatic colorectal cancer six years later, but he dies happy, knowing that Jake is safe.

A CHRONIC AUTOIMMUNE DISEASE

A 39-year-old woman presents to her GP with a two-month history of pain in her hands that is associated with swelling of her fingers and stiffness of her joints. The symptoms are worse in the morning. She has not had any previous serious illnesses.

On examination, the patient has symmetrical swelling of her fingers, particularly over the joints. No other joint deformity is present. No focal neurological signs are found.

The GP orders various blood tests and some X-rays. Among the blood tests is a request for an autoantibody profile.

Question 1

Autoantibody profiles are often requested in rheumatological disorders, vasculitis and liver disease. What antibodies are generally included and what is their significance?

Answer 1

The precise composition of an autoantibody profile will vary from hospital to hospital and the clinical case under investigation. The general purpose of the profile is to search for autoantibodies that are present in certain disease states and which help to indicate the diagnosis. Commonly featured antibodies include the following:

- Antineutrophil cytoplasmic antibodies (ANCA) may be either cANCA or pANCA in type, dependent on whether the pattern of staining on immunofluorescence is coarse, granular and cytoplasmic (cANCA) or perinuclear (pANCA). Both types of ANCA suggest a vasculitis. Wegener's granulomatosis is strongly associated with cANCA, which have a sensitivity of around 90 per cent and a specificity of approximately 95 per cent. A broader spectrum of conditions manifest pANCA, although they are traditionally grouped with microscopic polyarteritis.

- Antinuclear antibodies (ANA) are found in systemic lupus erythematosus (SLE), but are not specific. Despite the name, ANA target a variety of both nuclear and cytoplasmic antibodies.

- Anti-DNA are antibodies to double-stranded DNA and are considered to be specific for SLE.

- Anti-Sm is said to be specific for SLE.

- Anti-Ro (SSA) is associated with a variety of conditions, including Sjögren syndrome.

- Anti-La (SSB) partners anti-Ro.

- Anti-mitochondrial (AMA) are specific for primary biliary cirrhosis, but their utility is limited to investigating this diagnosis.

- Anti-liver kidney microsomes (anti-LKM), like AMA, are of use in liver diseases. There are several subtypes.

Question 2

The X-rays shown in Figure 38.1b could have come from this patient. What abnormalities are present?

Answer 2

The X-rays exhibit periarticular soft tissue swellings, periarticular osteopenia, erosion of the ulnar styloid and periarticular erosion.

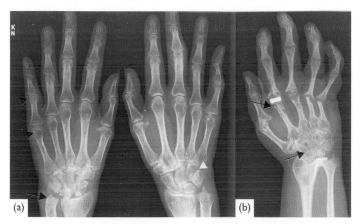

(a) (b)

Figure 38.1 (a) Early changes of rheumatoid arthritis with periarticular soft tissue swelling and periarticular osteopaenia (yellow arrow), erosion of the ulnar styloid (blue arrow) and periarticular erosions (red arrow). b) Late changes of rheumatoid arthritis with multiple carpal bone erosions and fusion (red arrow), a metacarpophalangeal joint prosthesis (blue arrow), and joint deformities.

A few days after having her X-rays, the patient notices a lump that has appeared in the olecranon region of her left elbow. She goes to see her GP who arranges for her to have an excision biopsy performed at the local day surgery unit. The histopathologist's microscopic description of the lesion is as follows (the conclusion to the report is discussed in the answer to question 6).

> *The specimen exhibits fibrous tissue in which there is a region of necrosis that is surrounded by a rim of fibrohistiocytic tissue in which foreign body type giant cells are abundant.*

Question 3

What are the causes of a polyarthropathy?

Answer 3

The causes can be quite diverse, but the following conditions should be considered:

- rheumatoid arthritis
- systemic lupus erythematosus
- psoriasis
- Reiter syndrome (usually an oligoarthropathy of larger joints)
- vasculitis
- gout
- scleroderma
- osteoarthritis.

This list is not exclusive.

Question 4

What two conditions are characteristically associated with nodules on the elbows?

Answer 4

This question is quite popular in exams. Nodules on the elbows should prompt consideration of rheumatoid arthritis and gout. Similarly, if asked to examine the hands, always seek to check the elbows as well.

Question 5

Is gout likely in this patient?

Answer 5

No. Gout is very unusual in premenopausal women. The presentation is also not typical as the arthritis in gout is usually very painful and episodic.

Question 6

What is the diagnosis and what basic pathological process underlies it?

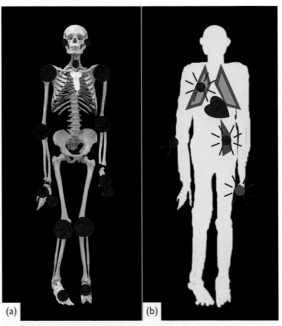

Figure 38.3 Sites of skeletal and non-skeletal involvement by rheumatoid arthritis. (a) Typical symmetrical polyarthritis includes cervical spine, the proximal interphalangeal joints of the hands and feet, knees, elbow, shoulder and temperomandibular joint. (b) About 25% of patients have non-tender red nodules in the skin, especially the elbow, forearm and hands, and elsewhere in the body, including heart valves, lung, spleen and other viscera. Severely affected patients may develop vasculitis which can cause gangrene of distal extremities and skin ulcers.

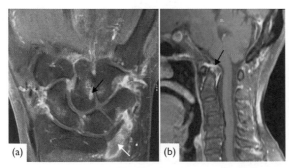

Figure 38.2 (a) Coronal MRI of hand with contrast showing synovitis (white arrow) and carpal bone erosion (black arrow). (b) Sagittal MRI post intravenous gadolinium showing enhancing rheumatoid pannus around the peg associated with erosion of the odontoid peg (arrow).

Answer 6

The patient has rheumatoid arthritis. Rheumatoid arthritis is an autoimmune disorder. The peak age at presentation is around 40–50 years and the disease is more common in women (M:F 1:3). Various patterns of disease exist, but the symmetrical polyarthritis affecting the hands and feet is typical. Rheumatoid arthritis is a destructive arthropathy, as in this patient. Around 20–30 per cent of patients have rheumatoid nodules, as this patient has on her elbow. The histopathologist's description is consistent with a rheumatoid nodule. The use of the word 'consistent' in a report is important to note as it implies that the pathologist's conclusion or the final diagnosis is dependent on data beyond that available from the specimen alone, for example the clinical context.

Question 7

Approximately 70 per cent of patients with rheumatoid arthritis have rheumatoid factor in their blood. This can be checked by a blood test. What is rheumatoid factor and what is its significance?

Answer 7

Rheumatoid factor is an autoantibody that is directed against the Fc portion of IgG. It is present in 5 per cent of the healthy population and also in a wide variety of rheumatological disorders, but if found in a patient with rheumatoid arthritis it indicates that the disease is likely to be more aggressive.

Question 8

What would a biopsy of the soft tissue of an affected joint show in rheumatoid arthritis?

Answer 8

The synovial cells proliferate in rheumatoid arthritis, causing the synovium to develop villiform folds. There is chronic inflammation that typically includes lymphoid follicles and plasma cells. Fibrinous material is present. There can be an increase in the number of small blood vessels.

The above changes are at first reversible, but if not treated they can progress to the generation of granulation tissue on the surface of the articular cartilage which is irreversible. The granulation tissue is referred to as pannus and interferes with the nutrition of the cartilage and causes degradation of the cartilage. The pannus can extend into the underlying bone, or across the joint to form adhesions, giving further joint destruction. Fibrosis of the granulation tissue can worsen joint adhesions.

Question 9

What other features may be encountered in rheumatoid arthritis?

Answer 9

Despite its name, rheumatoid arthritis is a multi-system disorder, mainly due to a combination of a vasculitic process and the development of rheumatoid nodules in various organs.

In addition to the arthritis of the limbs, spinal arthritis can develop and atlanto axial subluxation is a particularly serious complication.

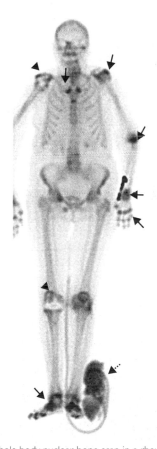

Figure 38.4 Whole body nuclear bone scan in a rheumatoid patient with involvement of the sternoclavicular joints, the elbow, the wrist, the metacarpophalangeal (MCP) joints, the shoulder, the knees and the feet (arrows). Note the right shoulder and knee prostheses (arrowheads) and the urinary catheter bag (dotted arrow).

The heart may show pericarditis. Conduction disturbances may be caused by rheumatoid nodules.

The lung can be affected by fibrosis, pneumonitis, rheumatoid nodules and pleuritis.

A neuropathy induced by rheumatoid vasculitis is rare, but the other inflammatory aspects of the disease can cause nerve compression or entrapment, or damage to the spinal cord.

Other than Sjögren syndrome, ocular disease is rare but includes episcleritis and scleritis.

Haematoreticular disease is usually seen in the form of Felty syndrome in which there is lymphadenopathy, splenomegaly, neutropenia and possibly anaemia and/or thrombocytopenia. Felty syndrome is uncommon (1–5 per cent).

Question 10

The patient is initially treated with non-steroidal anti-inflammatory agents. These provide disease control for a couple of years, but after this period the disease progresses and joint deformities develop and worsen. Various other agents are tried, including glucocorticoids and penicillamine, but it is found that the most effective agent in this patient is gold. Why are NSAIDs and steroids used in rheumatoid arthritis?

Answer 10

Given that rheumatoid arthritis is an autoimmune condition, treatments that are likely to be successful should have anti-inflammatory and/or immunosuppressant actions. As their name indicates, non-steroidal anti-inflammatory drugs (NSAIDs) damp down the process of inflammation. They achieve this by inhibiting the generation of the various inflammatory mediators that are produced by the arachidonic acid cascade. This also endows them with analgesic properties. In early rheumatoid arthritis, this combination of an analgesic effect and anti-inflammatory action can be quite effective. This is somewhat unusual for an autoimmune disease as they typically require more aggressive immunosuppression than NSAIDs.

Glucocorticoids are potent anti-inflammatory agents that are also immunosuppressants. If NSAIDs are ineffective in rheumatoid arthritis, steroids can be invoked.

The high doses of steroids that are required in many autoimmune diseases can induce Cushing syndrome and its numerous harmful features. Therefore, it can be desirable to find alternative agents which do not have such diverse adverse effects. One of the most commonly used is azathioprine. However, in rheumatoid arthritis, it has been found that both gold and penicillamine are effective, although they do not help in other autoimmune diseases.

Some patients with rheumatoid arthritis can be managed successfully with NSAIDs. Others have more resistant disease and multiple agents have to be tried before an effective drug is found.

Question 11

The patient's disease is well controlled on gold. Eighteen months after starting this line of treatment, she notices that her ankles and calves have become swollen, together with puffiness of her face and bloating of her abdomen. Examination reveals that the abdominal bloating is due to ascites. Her serum albumin is markedly reduced and her urinary protein excretion is 8 g per 24 hours. What has happened and is it related to her rheumatoid arthritis?

Answer 11

The patient has nephrotic syndrome. This is a renal disease in which there is protein loss through the glomerulus that amounts to at least 3.5 g/day (various figures are quoted around this range and some adopt a pragmatic definition that the nephrotic syndrome occurs when the level of proteinuria is sufficient to cause oedema). There are numerous causes of nephrotic syndrome, one of which is gold therapy.

SUMMARY

Rheumatoid arthritis is a multi-system autoimmune disorder of uncertain aetiology, in which the principle manifestation is arthritis. The underlying pathological process revolves around microvascular damage and defective T cell-mediated autoimmunity that involves complex cytokine cascades.

The differential diagnosis includes other causes of arthritis. The clinical presentation is frequently characteristic and the investigations aim to exclude other diagnoses, particularly through the use of autoantibodies.

Rheumatoid arthritis is a destructive arthropathy. Several characteristic deformities can result and these are due to combinations of joint destruction, subluxation, tendon disruption and derangement of the balance of actions of muscles at joints.

The severity of the disease is variable and in more aggressive cases assorted second-line agents can be necessary if NSAIDs fail. These second-line agents are associated with a variety of side-effects, some of them serious.

A 61-year-old man presents to accident and emergency with a 30-minute history of severe chest pain. The pain was of sudden onset while the man was at rest in his armchair, reading the newspaper. The pain is central and radiates up to the jaw. The patient mentions that he feels sick and generally unwell.

On examination, the man appears unwell and frightened and is pale and clammy. His pulse is 112/minute and regular. His blood pressure is 160/90 mmHg. The jugular venous pressure (JVP) is not raised. The apex beat is undisplaced but difficult to palpate; there are no heaves or thrills. The first and second heart sounds are normal. No added sounds or murmurs are heard. Bibasal crackles are present in the lungs, but examination of the respiratory system is otherwise unremarkable. The abdomen and nervous system are normal.

The man's ECG is shown in Figure 39.1.

Question 1

What is the diagnosis?

Answer 1

The man has an acute anterior myocardial infarction.

Question 2

What is the underlying pathological process?

Answer 2

Almost all myocardial infarctions are due to underlying atherosclerosis of the coronary arteries. Athcrosclerosis is discussed in more detail in Case 1, Intermittent chest pain (p. 2).

Question 3

What pathological process is happening in the myocardium?

Answer 3

As a result of the occlusion of its supplying coronary artery, the myocardium becomes ischaemic. If the ischaemia persists, irreversible cell death begins and the

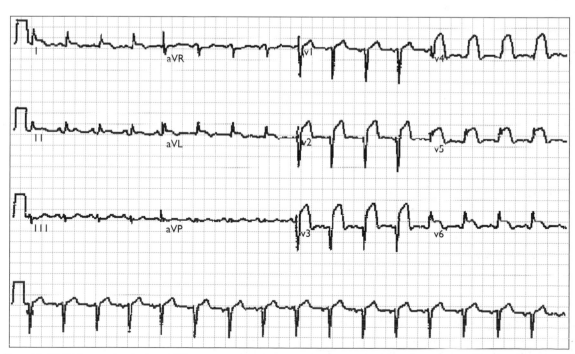

Figure 39.1 ECG from patient in Case 39. There is a raised ST segment, indicating an acute myocardial infarctiohn, hest seen in loads v2–6 (anterior leads).

process of coagulative necrosis occurs. This will result in an irreversible loss of the affected section of the myocardium, which will be replaced by fibrous scar tissue if the patient survives. The fibrous tissue lacks the contractile properties of the myocardium.

Question 4

Once the diagnosis of an acute myocardial infarction is made in this patient, he is given aspirin and thrombolysis. What is the rationale behind these treatments?

Answer 4

Thrombolytic therapy is usually in the form of streptokinase or recombinant tissue plasminogen activator (rTPA). These drugs stimulate the body's own thrombolytic pathways with the intention of breaking up the thrombus in the coronary artery and restoring circulation. This can limit the size of the infarction and if given early enough can be highly effective. Note that speed is of the essence in the administration of thrombolysis but that there are several contraindications to thrombolysis that must first be excluded.

Thrombolysis tends to assume the prominent and glamorous position in the acute treatment of a myocardial infarction (MI), such that the importance of the simpler aspirin is often wrongly underestimated. It should be remembered that in the initial papers that investigated thrombolysis the effect of aspirin alone on mortality was similar to that of thrombolysis.

Aspirin inhibits cyclo-oxygenase. This enzyme is vital in the metabolism of arachidonic acid. In platelets, its function is crucial to permit the synthesis of thromboxane A_2, a procoagulant agent. Aspirin therefore inhibits platelet-mediated thrombosis. In the context of a myocardial infarction, this can interrupt the development of the atherosclerotic thrombus and halt its extension, thereby reducing the size of the infarcted territory.

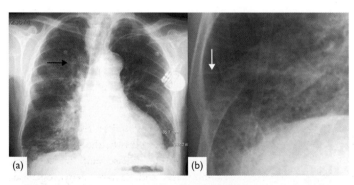

(a)   (b)

Figure 39.2 Heart failure in a patient following a myocardial infarct with cardiomegaly. (a) Distension of the upper lobe veins (arrow). (b) Interstitial lines at the base (arrow – so-called Kerley-B lines). These indicate septal/interstitial oedema.

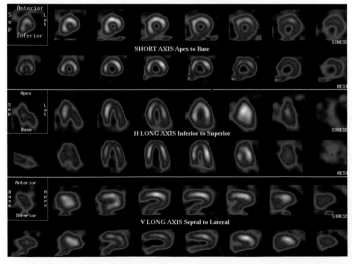

Figure 39.3 Nuclear medicine stress or myocardial perfusion test (see Figure 1.3). The relatively dark areas (arrows) show where myocardium is under- or not perfused. The images show underperfusion of the posterior or inferior wall of the left ventricle following maximal exercise (the top row in each projection) which remains underperfused at rest (the bottom row in each projection) in keeping with infarction.

Question 5

The patient is transferred to the coronary care unit. The introduction of coronary care units was one of the first measures to improve prognosis in acute MI. One of the facilities that they offer is constant ECG monitoring of the patients, supplemented by the provision of nursing staff trained in advance life support. Why is this important in acute MI?

Answer 5

One of the cellular consequences of ischaemia is the failure of Na^+/K^+-ATPase. In myocardial tissue, this is important in maintaining the negative electrical potential across the cell membrane. If this pump fails, the cell membrane depolarizes. In an electrically excitable tissue such as the myocardium, this can have serious consequences. Effective myocardial contraction depends upon the co-ordinated propagation of a depolarizing stimulus. Ischaemic, depolarized myocardium is susceptible to depolarizing spontaneously and acting as the focus for the generation of a tachyarrhythmia. Such arrhythmias can be fatal within minutes and in the case of ventricular fibrillation and ventricular tachycardia require immediate treatment with electrical defibrillation.

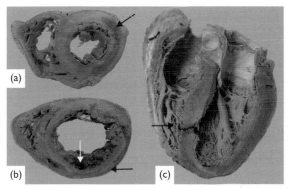

Figure 39.4 (a) Transverse slice through the left and right ventricles showing the bruised appearance of a recent myocardial infarction, about 2 days old, in the lateral aspect of the left ventricle. (b) Transverse section showing an established infarction, 3–4 days old, which is pale and softened (red arrow). The yellow arrow shows mural thrombus. (c) Vertical slice through a heart in which rupture of the interventricular septum is present. This infarct was around 5–7 days old, a time at which the damaged myocardium has been removed by macrophages, but fibrous scar tissue is incompletely developed, and the myocardium is soft and liable to rupture.

As well as tachyarrhythmias, serious bradycardias, including complete heart block, may occur if the damaged myocardium includes the conducting system. Inferior myocardial infarctions, caused by occlusion of the right coronary artery, are particularly prone to produce bradyarrhythmias because the right coronary artery supplies the sino-atrial and atrioventricular nodes.

Question 6

What drugs can be given to stop the complication of tachyarrhythmias?

Answer 6

Beta-blockers. These have a negative chronotropic, calming effect on myocardial contractility and depolarization and can stabilize the electrical activity of ischaemic myocardium.

Question 7

As part of his care, the patient has daily blood tests for the first few days. On the second day, he asks one of his doctors what the blood tests are for and is told that they are to help to assess the degree of damage to the patient's heart. To which blood test in particular is the doctor referring?

Answer 7

In broad terms, the doctor would be referring to cardiac enzymes. Until fairly recently, these involved the complexities of creatinine kinase and its isoforms, aspartate transaminase and lactate dehydrogenase. However, these have been superseded by troponin T. Nevertheless, the principle is the same for each enzyme and that is that damaged myocardium leaks its contents, some of which end up in the peripheral blood. The greater the volume of damaged myocardium, the greater the peak level of the cardiac enzyme(s) and the longer the duration for which it (they) will be elevated. Troponin T has the advantage over its predecessors of being specific for the myocardium and showing its initial rise earlier in the evolution of an MI.

Question 8

The patient becomes acquainted with the other patients in his bay, one of whom was admitted only a few hours after he was. The second patient has a history of asthma and is unable to receive beta-blockers.

The first patient is quite upset on the third day when the monitoring alarm goes off above his new friend's bed and, despite the immediate attention of the medical and nursing staff, the second patient dies. The following morning, the patient overhears the medical staff talking about a haemopericardium being found at the autopsy. How does this relate to the second patient's myocardial infarction, what are the related complications and what treatment can be given to try to prevent it?

Answer 8

An MI results in the death of the infarcted myocardium. The dead tissue is weaker than normal and is vulnerable to rupture. This can affect the free wall of the left ventricle, resulting in rupture of the ventricle and the expulsion of blood into the pericardial sac. The pericardial sac rapidly fills to capacity and compresses the venous return to the heart, resulting in tamponade. This complication is sudden and almost uniformly fatal (very rarely the rupture is locally sealed by the pericardium, leading to a false aneurysm).

Other than the free wall of the left ventricle, there can be rupture of the ventricular septum or a papillary muscle (yielding acute mitral regurgitation). Both of these complications impose a serious and potentially fatal haemodynamic disturbance on an already malfunctioning heart.

Beta-blockers reduce the incidence of all these types of rupture due to their negative inotropic effect on the heart.

Question 9

As a consequence of his MI, the patient finds himself started on several new drugs. These are explained to him by various staff. In addition to aspirin and beta-blockers, he is also prescribed an ACE inhibitor. Why?

Answer 9

The loss of myocardial tissue in an MI poses the danger of cardiac failure if sufficient ventricular mass is damaged. This is especially so in anterior MIs which frequently involve a significant volume of the left ventricle. ACE inhibitors have been found to reduce maladaptive changes that occur in the left ventricle in response to an MI, changes that exacerbate the tendency to cardiac failure.

As well as being long term, the cardiac failure in an MI may be acute and dramatic, typically if a large volume of myocardium becomes ischaemic and non-functioning. Prompt salvage with thrombolysis may help to save some of this myocardium.

Question 10

What other complications of MI can occur?

Answer 10

The damage to myocardial tissue induces an acute inflammatory response. This can involve the pericardium, resulting in pericarditis. Aspirin has anti-inflammatory properties and helps to control this inflammation.

Related to the acute inflammation is the formation of ventricular thrombus over the infarcted myocardium. The damaged myocardium releases tissue factor which triggers thrombosis. The defective cardiac contractions that may result from the MI can produce local turbulence which is also thrombogenic. This thrombus may be the source of emboli and these can cause complications such as a cerebrovascular accident. Aspirin's anti-thrombotic properties may be beneficial.

The damaged myocardium will be replaced by fibrous tissue. This can deform, leading to a left ventricular aneurysm. Thrombus may develop in the aneurysm and be a source of emboli. The presence of the aneurysm can impair cardiac function and conduction, leading to cardiac failure and/or arrhythmias.

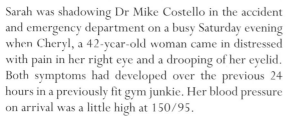

Sarah was shadowing Dr Mike Costello in the accident and emergency department on a busy Saturday evening when Cheryl, a 42-year-old woman came in distressed with pain in her right eye and a drooping of her eyelid. Both symptoms had developed over the previous 24 hours in a previously fit gym junkie. Her blood pressure on arrival was a little high at 150/95.

Mike asked Sarah to examine Cheryl's eye. Sarah noticed immediately that Cheryl had a drooping of her right eyelid (ptosis) which almost covered her eye. When Sarah raised the eyelid Cheryl complained of blurred and double vision. Sarah remarked that Cheryl's pupils were asymmetrical, with the right one being larger than the left. Mike looked increasingly concerned and asked Sarah to check on the light reflex. Cheryl's right pupil failed to constrict when Sarah shone a pen torch into the eye.

Question 1

Which anatomical structure do these symptoms and signs originate from?

Answer 1

The muscles of the orbit are supplied by cranial nerves III (oculomotor nerve), IV (trochlear nerve) and VI (abducens nerve). The III nerve supplies the eyelid muscle, papillary muscles and most of the extra-ocular muscles which enable movement of the globe.

Question 2

What are the causes of III nerve palsy?

Answer 2

- Ischaemic neuropathy (in diabetic patients)
- Head injury

- Cerebral artery aneurysm
- Inflammatory causes – meningitis, multiple sclerosis, sarcoidosis, vasculitis
- Tumours.

Mike took Sarah aside after performing a detailed neurological examination on the patient and explained that he was worried about a cerebral artery aneurysm causing Cheryl's symptoms. Cheryl was not a typical arteriopath, had not had a head injury and did not have any other neurological signs to suggest inflammatory or malignant conditions.

Sarah accompanied Cheryl to the CT scanner. Dr Sonia Jackson was the radiology registrar on call that night. She had brought her camp bed into the CT reporting room and was getting ready for a torrid night with a succession of head CTs on patients who had fallen over, had a stroke, got drunk or taken an overdose of recreational drugs. She perked up a little when Sarah told her about Cheryl. Sonia thought Cheryl should have a CT angiogram. This took five minutes after Cheryl was placed on the CT table and required an intravenous injection of iodinated contrast. Fifteen minutes later the processed images (Figures 40.1 and 40.2) appeared on Sonia's computer screen.

Within the hour Sonia's consultant Dr Milton Redman and the neurosurgeon on call, Mr Campbell, were poring over the images.

Question 3

What is an aneurysm and what types of aneurysms occur in the brain?

Answer 3

It is a localized dilatation in a blood vessel. This may be asymptomatic, press on adjacent structures such as

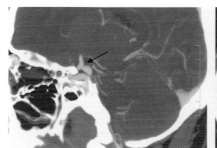
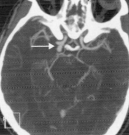

Figure 40.1 Processed sagittal and axial CT angiogram showing an aneurysm arising from the origin of the right posterior communicating artery (arrow). The oculomotor nerve passes close to the artery in the interpeduncular cistern as it leaves the midbrain and can therefore be compressed by an expanding aneurysm.

cranial nerves, become thrombosed and embolize distally or rupture resulting in a potentially catastrophic subarachnoid haemorrhage. Berry aneurysms develop because of a congenital defect in the media of the blood vessel at sites of bifurcation – usually in the vicinity of the circle of Willis – presenting in young or middle-aged adults. Microaneurysms of Charcot–Bouchard are small aneurysms more distally in the cerebral circulation which present with a cerebral bleed in elderly patients.

Rarely one sees post-infection mycotic aneurysms distally in the cerebral circulation.

Question 4

What are the other types of aneurysms?

Answer 4

Atheromatous aneurysms in the aorta are an important group because they require treatment before they rupture or close off the origins of their tributaries. They are usually fusiform (spindle-shaped) and are caused by a fairly widespread weakening of the wall secondary to atheroma deposition.

Weakening of the aortic media can also occur due to hypertension or inherited disorders of connective tissue, such as Marfan syndrome, and most commonly affects the arch of the aorta. These are not usually true dilated aneurysms but are often referred to as dissecting aneurysms because the blood dissects through a tear in the intima to track down between the middle and outer thirds of the media. This can result in a double-barrelled aorta, if the extra track ruptures back into the aorta, or death if it ruptures outwards.

The renal and mesenteric vessels can be damaged by arteritis, such as polyarteritis nodosa, producing aneurysms and local ischaemic damage.

Syphilis and other infections are rare causes of aneurysms.

Dr Redman and Mr Campbell talked at length with Cheryl and her husband who was with her at this stage. They explained that the aneurysm should be treated to stop a potential rupture. They felt that in Cheryl's case endovascular coiling would be effective in treating the aneurysm.

Question 5

What are the options for treating cerebral aneurysms?

Answer 5

Cerebral aneurysms can be treated surgically or with endovascular methods. Surgery involves a craniotomy and placing a clip across the neck of the aneurysm to exclude it from the circulation. Endovascular coiling involves placing a catheter in the femoral artery and

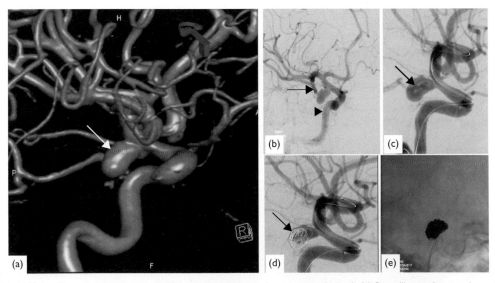

Figure 40.2 (a) Three-dimensional reprocessed CT image showing saccular aneurysm (arrow). (b) Precoiling angiogram via a catheter (arrowhead) placed in the cavernous internal carotid artery showing the anatomy of the aneurysm (thick arrow). (c) The tip of the microcatheter is in the aneurysm (arrow). (d) The detachable coils (arrow) are delivered into the aneurysm and effectively occlude the aneurysm at the end of the procedure. (e) Metallic coils in the aneurysm sac at the end of the procedure.

passing it through the aorta and carotid artery into the cranium. Microcatheters are used to enter the aneurysm. Detachable platinum coils are then delivered into the aneurysm sac eventually occluding the aneurysm with a combination of thrombus and coil. Eventually the aneurysm shrinks as it becomes excluded from the circulation. Coiling is associated with a more rapid recovery and shorter hospital stay than surgery and may also be associated with fewer potential complications. Not all aneurysms are suitable for coiling. A formally trained interventional neuroradiologist performs coiling

Early next morning Sarah reassured Cheryl as she lay nervously in the anaesthetic room of the interventional radiology suite. She was quickly anaesthetized and taken in. Sarah watched Dr Redman catheterize the aneurysm with a microcatheter and then deliver the coils into the sac.

A week later, Sarah went to visit Cheryl in the neurosurgical ward. Cheryl's ptosis had almost resolved and her double vision was improving. Her eye pain and headache had resolved 24 hours after her coiling procedure.

Question 6

What are the main types of cerebral haemorrhage?

Answer 6

The locations can be subdural, extradural, subarachnoid or intracerebral.

Subdural haematomas can be acute or chronic and most often occur because of rupture of the veins crossing the convexity of the cerebral hemispheres. This means that the pressure is fairly low compared with an arterial bleed and blood accumulates slowly and often without major symptoms unless the haemorrhage is large.

Extradural haematomas (epidural) generally follow skull fracture and especially rupture of the middle meningeal artery. They expand rapidly, compressing the underlying gyri and causing loss of consciousness.

Subarachnoid haemorrhages are most commonly due to rupture of a berry aneurysm or vascular malformation. They present with sudden severe headache (sometimes during strenuous activity   such as sexual

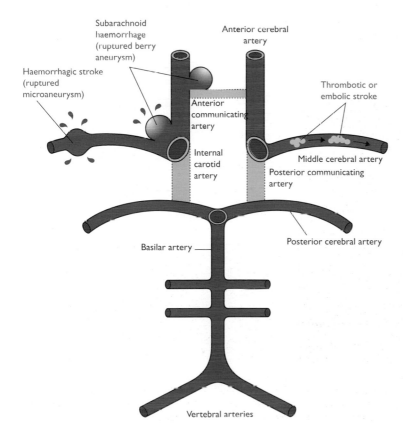

Figure 40.3 This diagram of the cerebral blood supply shows the circle of Willis and compares the sites at which haemorrhagic and thromboembolic strokes occur with the typical berry aneurysms.

intercourse), photophobia, neck stiffness and vomiting. Another common cause is head trauma. The blood in the subarachnoid spaces can irritate other vessels, leading to spasm and cerebral infarction. The hydrocephalus which can follow a subarachnoid haemorrhage contributes to raised intracranial pressure.

Intracerebral haemorrhages occur mostly in patients with hypertension who have microaneurysms located in the basal ganglia, pons and cerebellar cortex. Forty per cent will die in the first week.

Sarah was exhausted. She had not slept much in the last 48 hours because she was on an attachment to

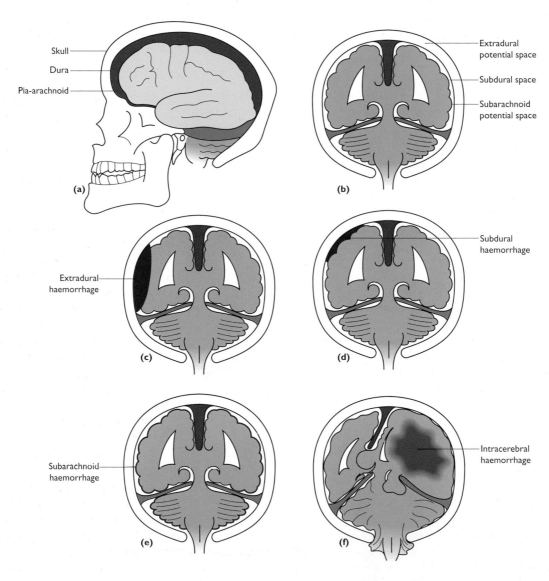

Figure 40.4 Sites of intracranial haemorrhage. (a,b) Normally the dura is densely adherent to the skull, thus trauma to the skull can lead to accumulation of blood between skull and dura (c). There is a relatively wide subdural space, criss-crossed with small vessels which bleed after trauma (d). The pia and arachnoid layers are effectively fused and a subarachnoid haemorrhage, commonly seen with ruptured berry aneurysm, leads to haemorrhage encasing the brain (e). This sometimes tracks along the optic nerves and is visible as a fluid level in the optic discs. Intracerebral haemorrhage behaves as a space-occupying lesion and can cause mid-line shift and coning (f).

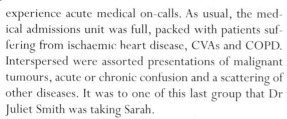

experience acute medical on-calls. As usual, the medical admissions unit was full, packed with patients suffering from ischaemic heart disease, CVAs and COPD. Interspersed were assorted presentations of malignant tumours, acute or chronic confusion and a scattering of other diseases. It was to one of this last group that Dr Juliet Smith was taking Sarah.

The bright yellow of the young female patient's sclerae was the first thing that Sarah noticed when she entered the cubicle. The striking blue of the patient's eyes perhaps provided a physiological contrast to the yellow.

Kara Ashcroft was 23 years old, employed in the advertising industry and had split up with her boyfriend of one year on Saturday afternoon after an acrimonious row. Distraught once her boyfriend had finally stormed out of her flat and the anger of the argument had given way to contemplation of its consequences, Kara had turned to a bottle of wine in her fridge for whatever comfort the best endeavours of her friends could not provide. By close to midnight, the bottle was empty, as were Kara's spirits. In a very dark moment, her reason clouded by the alcohol, she opened a new box of paracetamol tablets and swallowed all sixteen of them, plus another half dozen or so that were still in a loose blister panel from a partially finished box.

It was noon before Kara woke up on Sunday. Still miserable and far from refreshed despite her long sleep it required a few minutes before she was able to recall what she had done the previous night. Aghast at how she had reacted and certain that although she had seldom felt this low in her life before, she had no desire to die, she felt a sense of considerable relief that she was still alive and experiencing no ill-effects. Breathing a sigh of relief that her drunken misjudgement had not cost her her life, Kara spent a quiet Sunday at home, wondering how she would be moving on from the break up.

The fear in Kara's blue-in-yellow eyes told Sarah exactly what Kara must have thought when she woke up on Monday, just a few hours before Sarah and Dr Smith met her. Bright yellow, jaundiced sclerae would have shone back at her from her bathroom mirror, undeniable portents that her relief of Sunday was misplaced and that Kara was another of the sad list of people who had failed to appreciate how long a paracetamol overdose could take to wreak its malign effects.

Sarah was impressed with how Dr Smith handled Kara. She obtained the history of what had happened efficiently, but without obtrusive haste and still also ascertained Kara's state of mind at the time she took the overdose.

'Do you think she meant to kill herself?' Dr Smith asked of Sarah while they were filling in the labels on the assortment of blood samples that Dr Smith had taken from Kara.

'No. She basically said as much,' answered Sarah. 'She was drunk and very upset and got carried away.'

'That's what I think. It's a so-called parasuicide. They tend to occur in women rather than men, particularly younger women, often after emotionally traumatic events such as this and involve readily accessible, non-violent methods that don't require much planning. The doses of the drugs involved typically aren't that high and there's no real suicidal intent, like in Kara's case. Unfortunately, just because there's not any intent doesn't mean that the attempt won't have that effect, particularly where paracetamol's concerned.'

'Is she in that much danger, then?'

'Very possibly.' Dr Smith signed one request form and began filling in another. 'Obviously we've got a lot of blood tests here, but suppose you could only ask for one to see how badly damaged her liver was, which one box would you tick on these forms?'

'LFTs,' replied Sarah, 'to see how high her enzymes are and how much damage has already occurred.'

'That's close, but there's actually a better test of acute hepatic function. What we really need to know is how well her liver is functioning now. The enzymes don't tell you that. I'll give you a clue, it's not on the chemical pathology form.'

Sarah assumed a puzzled expression. 'Oh, the clotting,' she finally deduced.

'Exactly. The INR in particular is vital. It's like an honorary LFT and if you think the liver is up the spout, you should get an INR as well as the traditional LFTs. Clotting factors are one of the first things to suffer if the liver's struggling and the INR will pick that up. As you can see, we're also getting an FBC. If the clotting's deranged, you need to know whether the platelets are adequate and vice versa. Pre-existing anaemia won't help the situation either. U and Es check out the renal function. Has hepatorenal syndrome developed and how are the kidneys doing now, in case things deteriorate? You need the glucose because the liver has an important role in maintaining blood glucose and you should always have in the back of your mind the possibility of early diabetes being unmasked by an intercurrent illness. The last thing you need then is a diabetic crisis on top of everything else.

'Any idea why I've requested an aspirin as well as a paracetamol level?' added Dr Smith.

'Because people often take both. You can buy both of them over the counter. Sometimes patients might not tell, especially if they really are suicidal.'

'Yeah. Or if they forgot, for whatever reason, like they were drunk, or took something like a

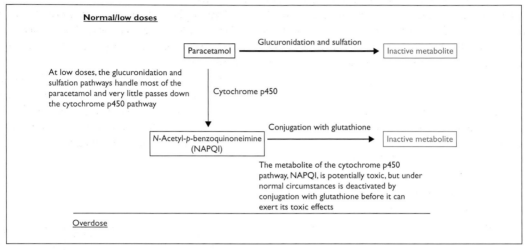

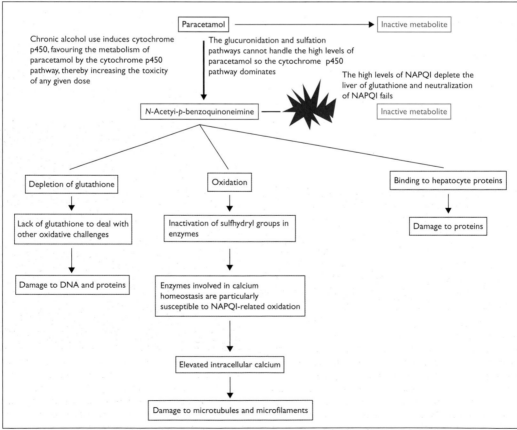

Figure 41.1 The metabolism of paracetamol.

benzodiazepine that affected their memory. It's also important to ask the lab to save the blood sample, in case any other drugs enter the equation later. Any other blood test that you'd do?'

'I can't think of any.'

'Blood gases. Acidosis is a bad feature. I need to contact the liver unit because she's presented a good 36 hours after taking the overdose, she's jaundiced and we should involve them sooner rather than later. Can you put the bloods in the airtube for me, please, then we can have a chat about the usual management of a paracetamol overdose.'

Sarah placed the blood samples and their forms into the appropriate bags, then sent them to the labs via the airtube delivery system.

'Right, the liver SpR [specialist registrar] is going to come down in a few minutes and take a look at her. You might want to follow this case through as I think you'll learn a lot from it, Sarah, but while you're waiting, what do you know about why paracetamol causes liver damage?'

The biochemistry lectures that had dealt with xenometabolism had been some time ago, but they had stuck in Sarah's mind, especially the parts about paracetamol. 'Normal doses of paracetamol aren't a problem. The liver glucuronidates them and they're inactivated. At higher doses, that pathway can't cope, so some of the paracetamol gets shunted through cytochrome p450 in hepatocytes. That produces a toxic metabolite which can damage hepatocyte DNA. However, that isn't normally a problem

because the liver puts a glutathione group on the toxic metabolite and neutralizes it.'

'So what goes wrong in an overdose?'

'The amount of the toxic metabolite swamps the liver's reserves of glutathione, so it doesn't get inactivated.'

'That's right. So how does that explain the antidote?'

'The antidote is acetylcysteine, which contains sulphur atoms and these replenish the liver's stocks of glutathione.'

'Okay. What about Kara's case could mean she's especially at risk, perhaps with a lower dose than under other circumstances? Don't forget that while the normal maximum daily total dose is 4 g, some people can run into trouble at just twice that, 8 g.'

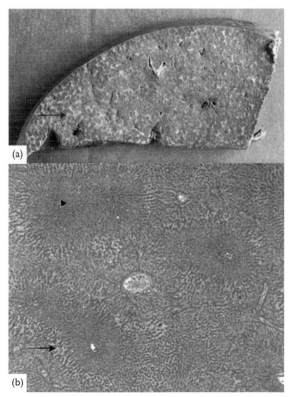

(a)

(b)

Figure 41.3 (a) Liver slice from a patient who died a few days after a paracetamol overdose. The pale areas are the necrotic liver. (b) Low-power photomicrograph showing collapse of the perivenular region (acinar zone 3) with haemorrhage, after liver cell necrosis (arrowhead). The surviving liver cells in the periportal zone 1 areas show a normal trabecular arrangement (thin arrow), surrounding dilated pale-appearing sinusoids.

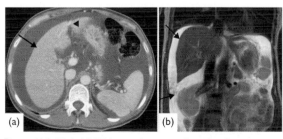

(a)   (b)

Figure 41.2 (a) Axial CT in a patient several weeks after a paracetamol overdose showing the development of portal venous hypertension (in the setting of chronic liver failure) with ascites (black arrow) and recanalization of the umbilical vein (arrowhead). The umbilical vein is normally only patent in fetal life and for a few months after. It carries oxygen from the placenta to the fetus. It reopens in cirrhosis and portal hypertension, shunting blood from the portal circulation to the systemic circulation. (b) Coronal T2 MRI in the same patient as in (a) showing the bright signal of the intraperitoneal fluid (arrows).

'The alcohol. It's an inducing agent so there's more cytochrome p450 around which means that the threshold at which paracetamol starts going down that pathway is reduced.'

'And in somebody who's an active alcoholic, which Kara doesn't seem to be, there's a danger that they'll have a poor diet which means that they start off with low glutathione reserves, as well as having induced enzymes. You can see what a mess that could be.'

Sarah nodded.

An hour later, Dr Uzma Zaman, the hepatology SpR had seen Kara and the labs were starting to return the results of the blood tests. The arterial blood gases were already known and were borderline acidotic. The INR was 2.3.

'We're going to take you up to the liver unit, Kara,' Dr Zaman explained. 'It's a special unit we have for dealing with people with damaged livers,' Dr Zaman had already told Kara what the problem was in relation to the injury caused by the paracetamol. 'We'll keep a very close eye on you there and do what's necessary. Is there anybody you'd like us to call for you?'

'My parents, I gave the number when I was first admitted,' said Kara. 'I'd really like them to be here now.'

'Of course. I'll take care of it. Do you want me to tell them what's happened?'

'I don't know,' answered Kara, who was a little tearful. 'I don't want to worry them, but it's too late for that and if they don't know what the problem is, they'll worry anyway.'

Dr Zaman nodded kindly. 'I'll tell them that you've had a bad reaction to some medication, which is true and then I can explain things properly when they arrive.'

'That would be good, thank you.'

Sarah accompanied Kara up to the liver unit where assorted lines and catheters were inserted and some more blood tests were taken. Sarah noticed how Kara bled a lot around the insertion sites and required a lot more pressure than usual to stop the bleeding. Her jaundice had deepened and she looked far from well. There was also not much urine in the catheter bag.

A little over an hour later, Kara's parents arrived. Understandably, it was a tearful few moments and Dr Zaman let them have them in privacy, before she took Kara's parents into an office to fill them in with the details, having earlier established Kara's permission to do this. Sarah waited with Kara during this time.

'I've really screwed up, haven't I?' Kara said to Sarah. It seemed to be more of a statement than a question.

Sarah was not sure what to say. Kara's observation was difficult to challenge in terms of her medical condition, but that was not what Kara needed to hear. 'You're in the right place now. Everybody knows what they're doing here. They'll sort you out, one way or another.'

'Can you stay with me, please?' asked Kara. 'All the doctors keep changing. First there was Dr Smith, now there's Dr Zaman who looks like she'll be around for a bit, but then there was the consultant and that male doctor when I came up. It's confusing, even though they've all been very nice. Now the nurses have changed shifts as well. I just need somebody around who knows what's going on who's been here from the start.'

'Of course.'

The afternoon slipped into the evening. Charts of vital signs and blood parameters all drew perturbed looks from anybody who studied them with a knowledgeable eye. The expressions were subtle and Kara would not have discerned them, but Sarah was used to doctors' reactions. By eight o'clock, the number of phone calls and other conversations that centred around Kara had increased in inverse proportion to Kara's level of alertness.

Dr Zaman beckoned Sarah over. Kara's parents were with her and Sarah had been talking to them for the last two hours, during which time Kara's participation had waned considerably.

'She needs a transplant,' Dr Zaman told Sarah. 'Her liver's too far gone for the parvolex to have had a chance and there's too much damage. All her parameters are going off and she's getting encephalopathic.'

'Just from 12 g of paracetamol?'

'That can be enough. I'm going to tell her parents. Would you mind being there? You seem to have developed a rapport with them and I'm going to be busy organizing things to spend much time once I've given them the news. They could do with a familiar face.'

'Sure.'

Kara's parents were predictably devastated when they heard the news. Kara was also distraught, although in her drowsy state, it was difficult to tell to what degree.

Dr Zaman spent the next half hour making a variety of phone calls, chasing results of various tissue typing analyses and notifying various people. The arrival of an anaesthetist gave Dr Zaman and Sarah the chance to have a talk about the transplant.

'Normally you'd have more time to work a transplant up,' began Dr Zaman, 'but Kara doesn't have that. She needs a new liver right now and she won't last more than a couple of days without one. As I'm sure you know, the body's immune system will recognize tissue from another person as foreign and reject it. What do you know about that and how we try to reduce the chances of that happening? I mean the things we do other than immunosuppression?'

Sarah recalled lectures from an immunologist who was not as funny as he thought he was, but nevertheless could convey material competently. 'You have to match basic blood groups. If you don't, the organ's rejected almost as soon as the blood supply is restored.'

'Yeah. Hyperacute rejection. It's a disaster and really shouldn't happen. Sarah's AB positive, so that's perhaps the first lucky break she's had. O negative is the universal donor and people often forget that AB positive is the universal recipient. Go on.'

'Then you have to match the HLA types. Somebody said they're like an ID card as far as transplants are concerned. If the donor organ doesn't have the right ID, T cells will recognize it and there'll be a T- and B-cell response.'

'That's acute rejection and happens in a few days after the transplant. You try to minimize it by HLA matching. The better the match, the less likely it is and the less heavy duty the immunosuppression you'll need. The strange thing is that you can often get away without this step in solid organ transplants. After that?'

'Chronic rejection. That's a more insidious process, maybe due to more minor tissue mismatches and inadequate immunosuppression. The donor organ fails slowly.'

'In a nutshell. And we've got just hours to sort all of that out for Kara. We got a head start by taking the bloods when she first came up to the unit. It wasn't exactly a feat of skill to know that a transplant was on

the cards, so we needed to get things rolling as soon as possible. Excuse me.' Dr Zaman's attention was summoned by one of her colleagues. She talked to them for a few moments then returned to Sarah.

'She's had another break, although it means that somebody else has just had some very bad news. There's a donor in Durham. The organ harvesting team are just leaving now. It's not a perfect match, but it's close enough for Kara and as she's now at the top of the liver transplant list, she'll be getting it. They'll be taking her to theatre before midnight. You might want to go along, if you're up for it. It'll be a long operation but it's not something you see every day and we're lucky that we actually have theatres here where you can see what's going on.'

Dr Zaman's prediction of the start time was accurate to 15 minutes. It was not only daylight but the start of another normal working day before Sarah emerged from the operating theatre. Kara's own liver had departed several hours ahead of her, swollen, red and congested and looking soft, friable and necrotic, ravaged by the paracetamol. The microscopic slides would be ready the next day, but Sarah's immediate thoughts were to return to the liver unit to keep her promise to Kara.

It was late afternoon before Kara regained some semblance of consciousness. The medical team were starting to speak in encouraging tones about Kara's prognosis and as she was almost out on her feet, Sarah decided that she would be no further use to anyone if she did not have some sleep.

Four days later Kara was looking much better. Her new liver had dealt with the accumulated problems left by her old, destroyed liver and her rehabilitation now centred around recovering from what was in itself major abdominal surgery.

PART 5

COMPLEX MANAGEMENT

A 67-year-old man is referred by his GP to the neurology outpatient department with a history of several weeks of weakness in his limbs. His previous medical history includes type 2 diabetes mellitus for 15 years. He is an ex-smoker, having smoked 15 cigarettes per day from the age of 21 to 55.

The patient does not think that the weakness came on suddenly. It is most noticeable in his hands.

On examination, the patient's first 11 cranial nerves are normal. However, he has fasciculations of his tongue.

Examination of the limbs reveals wasting of the small muscles of the hands. There are fasciculations in his right biceps, but the muscle bulk is preserved and his right biceps reflex is increased. Tone is elevated in his left forearm, but there is muscle wasting. Both patellar tendon reflexes are hyperreflexic, but his right quadriceps muscle group exhibits wasting. Clonus is elicited at the left ankle, but the left ankle reflex is absent and the left calf seems wasted.

The sensory examination is normal, as is co-ordination.

Question 1

What is unusual about the pattern of this man's motor signs?

Answer 1

Not only does the patient have mixed upper motor neurone (UMN) and lower motor neurone (LMN) features (see Case 11, Intermittent neurological signs (p.40)), but these mixed UMN and LMN features are present within the same muscle group. Furthermore, this mixture is found within several muscle groups.

For a patient with a single disease process, motor features tend to be either of the UMN or the LMN type, but not both. If both are present, either the patient has more than one disease, or a particular single disease becomes very likely.

Question 2

Is diabetes mellitus likely to be the explanation for his neurological features?

Answer 2

No. A sensory neuropathy tends to predominate in diabetes mellitus. In this patient, the features are exclusively motor. In addition, diabetic neuropathy affects the peripheral nerves only and this patient's UMN signs indicate an element of CNS disease.

Question 3

What single disease can affect both upper and lower motor neurones across several muscle groups, as in this case?

Answer 3

Motor neurone disease (MND). While it is important to be wary of dual pathology, or an unusual presentation of a systemic disease such as vasculitis, in a patient in whom the combination of UMN and LMN features is seen in three or more muscle groups, in the absence of sensory features, motor neurone disease is very likely.

Question 4

What patterns of features can be encountered in this disease?

Answer 4

Three main patterns are seen, depending on where in the motor nervous system the disease process dominates. Overlap can occur.

- Amyotrophic lateral sclerosis dominates in the corticospinal tract, giving mainly UMN features.
- Progressive muscular atrophy affects the anterior horn cells, yielding LMN signs.
- Bulbar palsy focuses on the cranial nerves and the muscles of the head and throat.

Note that the extraocular muscles are virtually never affected in MND.

Question 5

What is the basic pathology of the disease?

Answer 5

As the name implies, the disease shows loss of motor neurones in the corticospinal tract and the anterior horn of the spinal cord. These pathways become atrophic and smaller.

The pathogenesis is uncertain. Most cases are acquired. Inherited cases tend to have an earlier age of onset and a much longer survival. Current theories

Pyramidal cells in primary motor cortex
Final output of the brain to the motor neurones in the spinal cord
Receive projections from basal ganglia, cerebellum, higher motor regions and other higher regions
Also known as upper motor neurones. Much of their basal activity is inhibitory and serves to suppress primitive reflexes that operate at a subcortical and spinal level and are unwanted in the presence of higher motor skills

Basal ganglia
Receive projections from various sensory pathways and brain regions and assist with the development of motor functions. Project to the primary motor cortex to influence the output of this region. Precise functions remain to be elucidated Disease states are characterized by increased tone (rigidity), abnormal movements (e.g. tremor, chorea, athetosis) and bradykinesia, but not paralysis of voluntary movement.

Other sensory fibres
Assorted somatosensory fibres such as pressure, pain, fine touch and crude touch, project to the cerebral cortex and the cerebellum and are integrated to assist in the development of optimal motor output signals

Cerebellum
Receives sensory information from proprioreceptors and other somatosensory fibres. Also receives input from vestibular system. Sends fibres to and receives them from the primary motor cortex.
Integrates data from these various sources to coordinate movement and modify the activity of the primary motor cortex.
Disease states are characterized by impaired coordination, either of basic motor functions such as balance and eye movements and/or complex skilled movements (including speech)

Muscle spindle
Measures the degree of stretch in a muscle and tendon.
Serves to help to maintain the resting state of tone of the muscle and is essential to the spinal stretch reflex.
Provides crucial proprioreceptive information for co-indination

Sensory data going to brain

Skeletal muscle fibre

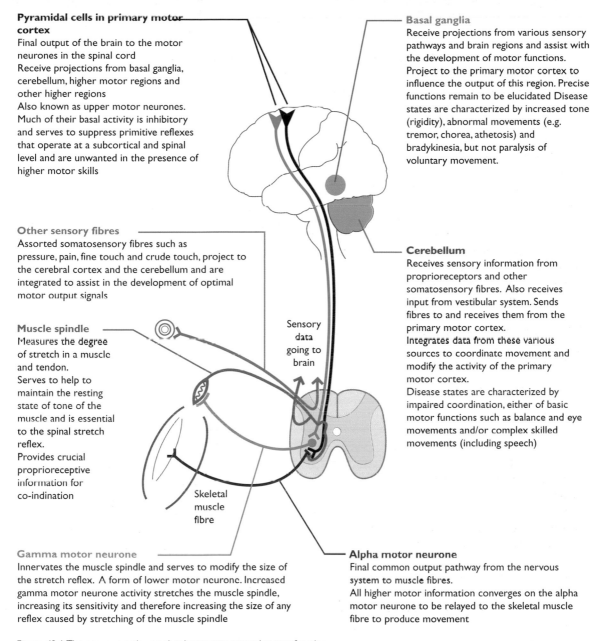

Gamma motor neurone
Innervates the muscle spindle and serves to modify the size of the stretch reflex. A form of lower motor neurone. Increased gamma motor neurone activity stretches the muscle spindle, increasing its sensitivity and therefore increasing the size of any reflex caused by stretching of the muscle spindle

Alpha motor neurone
Final common output pathway from the nervous system to muscle fibres.
All higher motor information converges on the alpha motor neurone to be relayed to the skeletal muscle fibre to produce movement

Figure 42.1 The nervous pathways that interact to control motor function.

revolve around excitotoxicity, in which excitatory amino acid neurotransmitters are believed to mediate cell death by causing an excessive influx of calcium ions through ion channels. Free radicals are also implicated.

Question 6

What is the usual prognosis?

Answer 6

Motor neurone disease is typically relentlessly progressive. Patients tend to die within three years.

Question 7

The patient is given the diagnosis. Eighteen months later, he is admitted to hospital from a nursing home suffering from a fever. Examination discloses that he has 4 × 3 cm ulcers over both heels and a 8 × 6 cm ulcer over his sacrum. All three ulcers are deep. That over his right heel exposes tendons. Deep soft tissues are observed in the sacral lesion. At this point in his disease, the patient has been immobile for three months and has difficulty in swallowing. He has marked wasting of all four limbs. What is the diagnosis of his skin lesions?

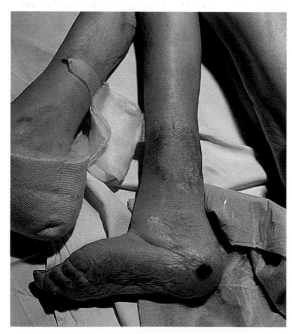

Figure 42.2 Poor blood supply, oedema of the lower limbs, poor nutrition and infection may all contribute to the failure to heal of a pressure sore in a bed-ridden patient.

Answer 7

The patient has pressure sores. The heels and sacrum are typical locations for pressure sores and the patient's condition places him at great risk of these lesions (see Figure 42.2).

Question 8

Why is the patient at risk of this complication?

Answer 8

Pressure sores arise in patients who have decreased mobility. Constant pressure on weight-bearing areas, typically the sacrum and heels in somebody lying in bed, can lead to breakdown of the skin. If the problem persists, the ulcer becomes deeper. In extreme cases, the ulcer can extend down to bone.

The development of pressure sores becomes more likely if certain risk factors are present. These relate to wound healing.

Question 9

What factors are necessary for good wound healing?

Answer 9

Wound healing can be considered to be analogous to a construction site project. Raw materials are necessary to form the new structure. Adequate transportation networks must be in place to bring these raw materials to the construction site. The damaged structure must be cleared away. Vandals must be stopped from entering the site and disrupting the process. The problem which caused the damage in the first place must be prevented from recurring.

In wound healing, this analogy equates to adequate nutrition to provide the energy and proteins necessary for generating new tissue. Good blood flow is essential to deliver nutrients and oxygen to the tissue, as well as for transporting breakdown products away. The immune system is necessary for preventing infection of the wound and for clearing away debris.

Question 10

Given the factors necessary for wound healing, why might this patient be at particular risk of pressure sores?

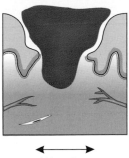
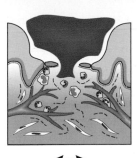
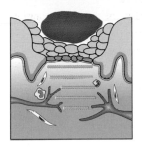
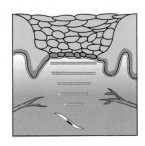

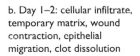

Wound gap

a. Fibrin clot

Wound gap

b. Day 1–2: cellular infiltrate, temporary matrix, wound contraction, epithelial migration, clot dissolution

c. Day 3–4: surface intact, new basement membrane, definitive matrix

d. Day 5: scar

Figure 42.3 Bedsores illustrate the principle of healing by secondary intention, which occurs when much tissue has been lost and leads to appreciable scar formation. By contrast a surgical incision, in which little damage is caused to dermal and subcutaneous tissues and in which the sides can be brought together by suturing, heals with virtually no scarring.

Answer 10

The patient has a history of smoking and diabetes mellitus. Both of these conditions can produce microvascular insufficiency and this can impair would healing, especially at a distal site such as the heel.

The patient's MND-related dysphagia will cause problems with maintaining an adequate nutritional intake.

As well as being the cause of the immobility which underlies the pressure sores, the patient's MND has also produced muscle wasting. This loss of muscle padding renders the skin more susceptible to the pressure effects related to the underlying bone.

Immobility can also cause problems with personal hygiene, including those related to the excretion of urine and faeces. Prolonged contact of the skin to these agents can facilitate the development of pressure sores.

Question 11

What steps can be taken to reduce the chance of developing pressure sores?

Answer 11

Prevention is the key strategy in handling pressure sores. A vital step is recognizing which patients are at risk and this is derived from an understanding of the basic pathology of wound healing.

Patients at risk can be nursed on special mattresses which redistribute the weight-bearing load by varying inflation and deflation of different compartments of the mattress. Help in moving and turning the patient frequently is important, as is assisting the patient in maintaining their personal hygiene. Diet should be adequate and provided in a manner that the patient can effectively eat and absorb. Scrupulous surveillance of pressure areas is also essential.

A 53-year-old woman presents to accident and emergency with a rapidly progressive, painful skin rash. The rash commenced the previous day with widespread erythema that initially affected the patient's arms and legs. As the patient had been doing some gardening during the sunny day before, she initially attributed it to the sun and irritation by plant sap. However, the rash rapidly spread and became tender. Shortly after this, blisters began to form and, a few hours prior to her arrival at hospital, her skin started to slough off from some of the affected areas. By the time of her attendance at accident and emergency, the extent of this sloughing had become much worse.

Her previous medical history is largely unremarkable, although she had begun taking antibiotics for a urinary tract infection two days before the rash appeared.

On examination, the patient is tachycardic and appears dehydrated. Large areas of the superficial layers of her skin have been lost. In addition, she has numerous blisters and widespread erythema. A few more discrete lesions are revealed by close inspection and these consist of concentric rings of erythema that resemble a target.

Question 1

What is the likely diagnosis?

Answer 1

Toxic epidermal necrolysis.

The targetoid lesions are a characteristic feature of toxic epidermal necrolysis, as is the widespread erythema and skin loss.

Question 2

A skin biopsy is performed and confirms the clinical impression. What basic process is happening in the skin in this disease?

Answer 2

In toxic epidermal necrolysis, the epidermis is targeted by a lymphocyte-based autoimmune reaction. The direct cytotoxic action of T lymphocytes, in conjunction with the effects of cytokines such as tumour necrosis factor, destroys the keratinocytes of the epidermis. The initial stage of erythema reflects the beginning of this inflammatory reaction. The formation of blisters denotes damage to the keratinocytes, in particular the adhesion of the basal layer of the epidermis to the underlying dermis. Breakage of this adhesion and loss of cohesion between keratinocytes, together with local oedema also induced by the inflammation permits the epidermis to separate from the dermis and form a blister. As the process continues, the inflammation completes the destruction of the keratinocytes that form the blister and the dead epidermis sloughs off, being no longer adequately anchored to the underlying dermis.

Question 3

How could a person's immune system come to mount such a powerful response against their own skin?

Answer 3

As far as the magnitude of the response is concerned, the function of the immune system is to destroy anything it recognizes as foreign. Therefore, while the effects of this are potentially catastrophic in toxic epidermal necrolysis, the degree of the immune reaction is consistent with the role of the immune system, albeit that the target identification is aberrant.

The mechanisms by which the immune system's ability to separate self from foreign is deranged in toxic epidermal necrolysis are not established in precise detail. However, it is believed that there is some sort of initiating trigger, typically either an infection or a drug, which either causes cross-reactivity between the trigger and the antigenic properties of the skin, or modifies the antigenicity of the skin such that it now appears foreign to the immune system. In the case of drug-induced

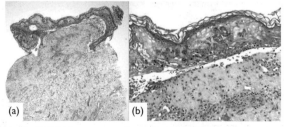

(a)   (b)

Figure 43.1 (a) Low-power view of a skin biopsy that displays toxic epidermal necrolysis. The epidermis has separated from the dermis. There is little remaining inflammation, possibly because the immune system has destroyed its target and moved on. (b) Higher power view to demonstrate the epidermal necrosis. Most of the keratinocytes are ghost cells which have lost their nuclei.

toxic epidermal necrolysis, certain metabolites of the drug can act as haptens on epidermal molecules and mislead the immune system.

Question 4

Toxic epidermal necrolysis is rare, yet some of the viral infections that can cause it are not. Similarly, many of the drugs that can precipitate the condition are in common use. How could toxic epidermal necrolysis be only a rare complication of common events?

Answer 4

The precise details for this process are also not fully elucidated, but in general terms, the phenomenon relates to genetic variation. Different HLA phenotypes have different susceptibilities to autoimmune disease, for example, the strong association between HLA-B27 and ankylosing spondylitis, or the tendency for people with organ-specific autoimmune diseases to be HLA DR3- or DR4-positive. In toxic epidermal necrolysis, certain HLA phenotypes and other aspects of immune function that demonstrate genetic polymorphism may render the individual more vulnerable to developing an aberrant immune response against the epidermis, should an appropriate precipitating event occur.

In parallel to genetic variation in the immune system is the polymorphism of xenometabolism. Different people will metabolize some drugs at different rates and by different pathways. This leads to the accumulation of different metabolites at different concentrations. Some of these metabolites may be able to act as haptens that could trigger toxic epidermal necrolysis.

The element of coincidence is also important. A person may have the immune constituents that render them susceptible to toxic epidermal necrolysis, but never meet a trigger that will precipitate the process, so

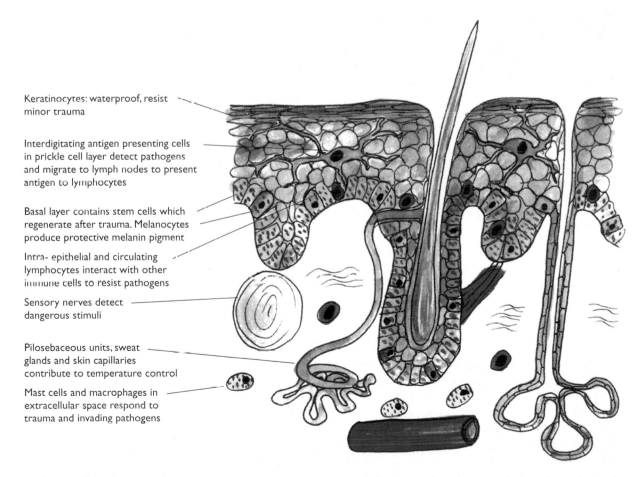

Keratinocytes: waterproof, resist minor trauma

Interdigitating antigen presenting cells in prickle cell layer detect pathogens and migrate to lymph nodes to present antigen to lymphocytes

Basal layer contains stem cells which regenerate after trauma. Melanocytes produce protective melanin pigment

Intra- epithelial and circulating lymphocytes interact with other immune cells to resist pathogens

Sensory nerves detect dangerous stimuli

Pilosebaceous units, sweat glands and skin capillaries contribute to temperature control

Mast cells and macrophages in extracellular space respond to trauma and invading pathogens

Figure 43.2 Skin has many roles.

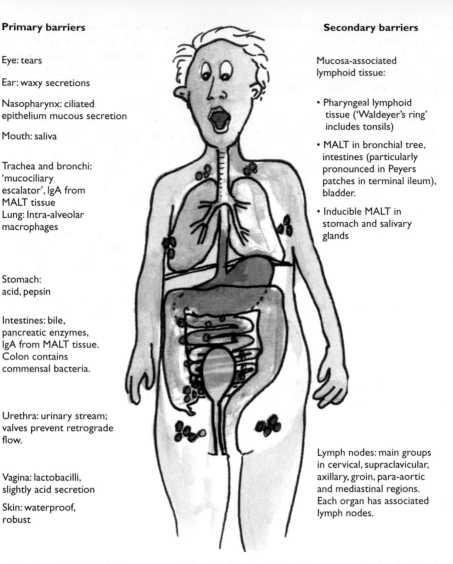

Primary barriers

Eye: tears

Ear: waxy secretions

Nasopharynx: ciliated
epithelium mucous secretion

Mouth: saliva

Trachea and bronchi:
'mucociliary
escalator', IgA from
MALT tissue
Lung: Intra-alveolar
macrophages

Stomach:
acid, pepsin

Intestines: bile,
pancreatic enzymes,
IgA from MALT tissue.
Colon contains
commensal bacteria.

Urethra: urinary stream;
valves prevent retrograde
flow.

Vagina: lactobacilli,
slightly acid secretion

Skin: waterproof,
robust

Secondary barriers

Mucosa-associated
lymphoid tissue:

• Pharyngeal lymphoid
  tissue ('Waldeyer's ring'
  includes tonsils)

• MALT in bronchial tree,
  intestines (particularly
  pronounced in Peyers
  patches in terminal ileum),
  bladder.

• Inducible MALT in
  stomach and salivary
  glands

Lymph nodes: main groups
in cervical, supraclavicular,
axillary, groin, para-aortic
and mediastinal regions.
Each organ has associated
lymph nodes.

Figure 43.3 Natural barriers to infection: the importance of skin and other epithelial surfaces as protective barriers is only really appreciated once they have been breached.

the disease never happens. Similarly, a person might have the metabolic pathways that allow them to generate the harmful haptens, but their immune system may be resistant to being fooled by them and toxic epidermal necrolysis never supervenes.

Question 5

Returning to the patient, what problems is she likely to face as a consequence of large parts of her epidermis being lost?

Answer 5

Toxic epidermal necrolysis is a life-threatening condition that emphasizes some of the functions of the skin.

The skin is a waterproof barrier. When it is disrupted over a large area, the volume of water lost through the skin is greatly increased because this waterproofing is compromised and the underlying tissues become exposed to the air. Thus, regulating fluid balance can be challenging.

The skin is also a barrier to infection and can be considered to be the outermost element of the innate immune system. When the skin is breached, microorganisms have a means of access to the body that would not normally be available to them. In toxic epidermal necrolysis, this breach is large.

As well as protecting against water loss, the skin is important in reducing heat loss (as well as facilitating heat loss when necessary). This thermoregulatory capacity of the skin is severely disrupted in toxic epidermal necrolysis and the patient can have difficulty in maintaining their core temperature.

Exposure of large areas of the subepidermal tissues is painful and providing adequate analgesia is vital.

Question 6

What other diseases could be present that would further complicate the management of a patient with toxic epidermal necrolysis?

Answer 6

The problem of managing a patient's fluid balance becomes even greater if they have co-existing cardiovascular disease. Such patients are less able to tolerate fluid overload and the balance between ensuring that the patient does not become fluid depleted, yet does not suffer cardiac failure from fluid overload can be delicate.

Toxic epidermal necrolysis places the body under considerable stress. Any stressful intercurrent illness can derange previously stable control of diabetes mellitus. Patients with type 2 diabetes may temporarily require insulin and those with type 1 diabetes may require significant changes to their normal dose. Sliding scale regimes usually provide the best solution to this problem.

Addison's disease is less common than diabetes mellitus and sometimes goes undiagnosed for some time. However, a patient who is coping reasonably well with subclinical Addison's disease, or who is a known patient controlled on oral replacement therapy may suffer an Addisonian crisis when the stress of the new illness overwhelms their failing adrenal corticosteroid system.

A 29-year-old man is walking in the park with his friends when he suddenly collapses and is witnessed to lose control of his bowels and begin generalized shaking of all of his limbs. This episode lasts for three minutes, during which time he is unresponsive. After the episode stops spontaneously, the man is in a deep sleep. An ambulance is called and the man is taken to the accident and emergency department of the local hospital.

On arrival at accident and emergency, it transpires that the man has no history of seizures and has been previously fit and well, although he does mention that he has had a dry cough for the past few days and has felt short of breath on exertion, as well as having headaches. He had attributed this to a 'bad cold with a touch of bronchitis'.

No abnormality is found on examination.

The patient's full blood count, urea and electrolytes and liver function tests are normal. The chest X-ray reveals subtle shadowing in the lung fields radiating out from both hila in a 'batwing' distribution. An urgent brain CT scan is performed and shows an enhancing mass in the right frontal lobe. Extension of the scan beyond the originally intended region does not discover any other mass lesions.

A neurosurgical and oncological opinion is obtained and the patient undergoes a biopsy of the cerebral lesion. The histopathology report gives a diagnosis of a diffuse large B cell lymphoma. A chest opinion has also been sought and it has been determined that while the patient has normal oxygen saturations at rest, he is susceptible to marked desaturation on exertion. A bronchoscopy is undertaken and includes a brochoalveolar lavage (BAL).

Question I

What abnormality is the BAL likely to show?

Answer I

The diagnosis of *Pneumocystis carinii* pneumonia (PCP) is the anticipated finding in the fluid obtained from the BAL.

The clinical and radiological picture of the patient's respiratory problem is in itself suggestive of PCP. Desaturation on exertion is characteristic, in the appropriate clinical setting, as is the 'batwing' pattern on chest X-ray (although other conditions, such as uraemia, can have a similar distribution of radiological changes). The cough in PCP is typically dry. However, *Pneumocystis carinii* is not a normal cause of pneumonia and requires an appropriate context in which to suspect it.

Question 2

Which group of patients is susceptible to PCP?

Answer 2

Patients who have defective cell-mediated immunity.

Question 3

Are the any reasons to suspect that the patient has defective cell-mediated immunity (other than the presence of PCP)?

Answer 3

The patient has a cerebral lymphoma. According to the CT, this seems to be a primary CNS lymphoma as there is no CT evidence of lymphoma outside the brain. Primary CNS lymphoma is a characteristic finding in a particular condition in which there is defective cell-mediated immunity.

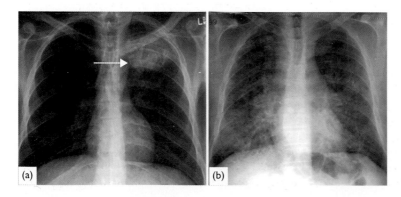

Figure 44.1 (a) Chest X-ray from a 37-year-old male patient with HIV and *Mycobacterium avium intracellulare* (MAI) infection (arrow). (b) Chest X-ray from a 27-year-old male patient with HIV showing diffuse bilateral lung infiltrates – *Pneumocystis carinii* pneumonia (PCP).

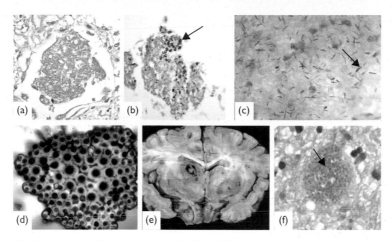

Figure 44.2 (a) H&E and (b) Grocott show *Pneumocystis carinii* (PCP) and (c) shows *Mycobacterium avium intracellulare* (MAI). These are two commonly encountered organisms in HIV/AIDS patients with pneumonia. However, tuberculosis is the major global cause of death in HIV/AIDS. (d) *Cryptococcus* and (e,f) *Toxoplasmosis* are two of the most common infective intracerebral lesions found in HIV/AIDS.

Question 4

In which disease is a primary CNS lymphoma a characteristic finding?

Answer 4

In a patient who has human immunodeficiency virus (HIV) infection, a primary CNS lymphoma is an 'AIDS-defining illness', as is PCP.

The progression from the presentation, through the selection of the specific investigations, to the diagnosis of acquired immune deficiency syndrome (AIDS) in this patient may seem abrupt, but there are certain important points.

The patient has no previous history of seizures. While approximately 3 per cent of the population are said to experience a seizure at some point in their life, the new onset of primary epilepsy in an adult should be viewed with caution until an underlying cause for seizures is excluded. A common secondary cause of a seizure is a mass lesion. In isolation, the patient's history of a headache could have numerous causes. However, when combined with a seizure, the emphasis shifts to excluding a mass lesion.

Under ordinary circumstances, the patient's interpretation of his dry cough could well be plausible. However, the chest X-ray findings are not congruent and as discussed above, do raise a certain possibility.

When the existence of a CNS mass lesion and a respiratory problem that could be PCP are combined, HIV/AIDS enters the differential. The biopsy finding of a lymphoma greatly strengthens this suspicion.

Question 5

How does the HIV virus cause immunosuppression?

Answer 5

The HIV virus infects and kills the CD4 subset of T lymphocytes. These are the helper T cells and have a central function in the regulation of many aspects of the immune system. If the CD4 T cell population is depleted, the immune system's ability to organize its response against various types of infection is lost. Therefore, while the other individual components of the immune system may remain functional, they cannot operate in a co-ordinated fashion and this is enough to hamper the efficacy of the immune response.

Question 6

To what sorts of infection are people with defective T cell-mediated immunity susceptible and why?

Answer 6

The T cell response is particularly useful for dealing with intracellular organisms, such as viruses, mycobacteria and some fungi. This relates to the ability of cytotoxic T cells to destroy infected cells. However, this destructive ability of cytotoxic T cells is a weapon that must be tightly regulated to prevent it from activating inappropri-

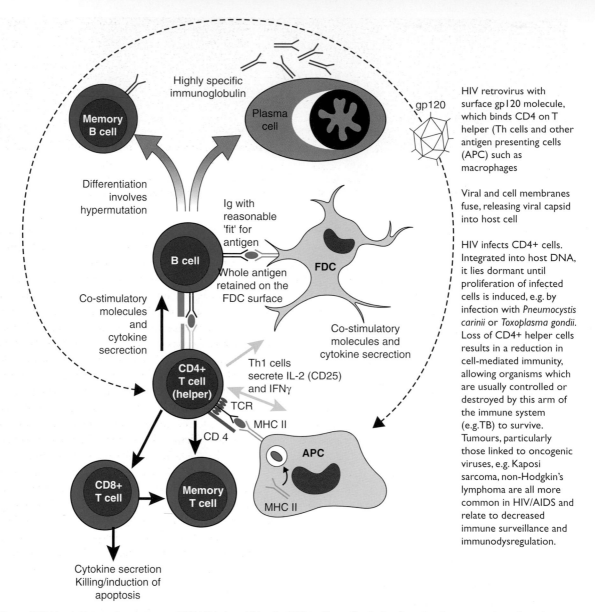

Figure 44.3 Normal interactions between CD4+ T helper (Th) cells, CD8+ effector T cells, B cells and antigen-presenting cells, such as macrophages are interfered with by HIV infection. The cells co-ordinate the acquired cell-mediated and humoral immune responses.

ately. T helper cells are important in giving cytotoxic T cells permission to strike. Therefore, if the helper T cells are crippled, the cytotoxic response is also hamstrung.

Question 7

Why is the immune response to bacterial infection better preserved and are there any problems with this aspect of the immune system in HIV/AIDS?

Answer 7

As extracellular organisms, bacteria are ideal targets for antibodies and therefore fall within the province of the B lymphocyte–plasma cell system. B lymphocytes can be stimulated directly by their cognate antigen without the need for T cells to assist them and thus bacterial infections can still be addressed if T cell function is defective. However, the B cell response is more

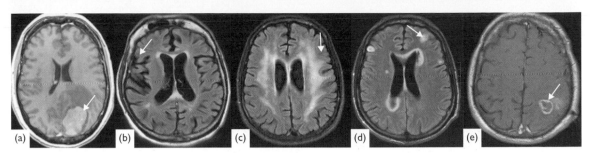

Figure 44.4 MRI scans from HIV-positive patients. (a) Enhancing left occipital mass (arrow) in a 53-year-old patient with cerebral lymphoma. (b,c) HIV encephalitis in a 37-year-old man with cortical atrophy (b, arrow) and 'bright' inflammatory white matter changes (c, arrow). (d) From 47-year-old man with HIV and cerebral cryptococcosis (arrow). (e) Cerebral toxoplasmosis in a 42-year-old man.

complex. Activated helper T cells can also activate B cells, thereby augmenting the B cell response. Furthermore, B cells are dependent on T cells to switch their immunoglobulin class from IgM to IgG or IgA. The availability of appropriate immunoglobulin sub-classes is vital to provide an optimal response. T cells also assist B cells in hypermutating their immunoglobulin to provide the best specificity for the target antigen, as well as allowing the generation of memory B cells. Therefore, if there is a problem with T helper cells, B cell performance is suboptimal.

In addition to the impairment of the B cell response in HIV/AIDS, there can be a polyclonal increase in immunoglobulins. This also reflects dysregulation of B cell activity.

Question 8

What term is employed for the infections that characterize HIV/AIDS and other diseases of immunocompromisation?

Answer 8

Opportunistic infections. These are infections by organisms that are normally not able to cause an infection in a healthy person. However, when the immune system becomes defective, they are able to take advantage of this weakness.

Question 9

Why are certain types of tumour more common in HIV/AIDS?

Answer 9

The immune system has a role in suppressing neoplasia. Neoplastic cells can express altered proteins on their cell surfaces as a result of the mutations that have transformed them into neoplastic cells. The immune system, especially T cells and NK cells, can recognize these proteins and attempt to remove the cells.

High-grade B cell lymphomas are among the most common malignancies in HIV/AIDS. As mentioned above, the regulation of B cell function is already disordered by the depletion of the helper T cell population. This situation becomes exacerbated by the ability of the Epstein–Barr virus (EBV) to intercalate itself into the DNA of B cells and overdrive their proliferation. Loss of the T cell response to EBV in HIV/AIDS permits infected B cells to proliferate aberrantly (the B cells may have been infected many years prior to the onset of HIV/AIDS and have behaved normally due to adequate regulation by the helper T cell system during this interval). In some cases, this is accompanied by the accrual of mutations that culminate in malignant transformation.

Interestingly, one of the other characteristic malignant tumours of HIV/AIDS, Kaposi's sarcoma, is intimately related to human herpes virus type 8. Furthermore, cervical carcinoma, which is dependent on the human papilloma virus, is an AIDS-defining illness in a patient known to have HIV.

Question 10

What specific treatment is given in HIV/AIDS?

Answer 10

Highly active antiretroviral therapy (HAART). HAART aims to reduce the viral load. This allows the CD4 T lymphocyte population to increase, restoring immuno-competence. This can be very helpful in tackling both opportunistic infections and opportunistic malignancies, although specific antimicrobial and oncological therapy will still be required.

A 20-year-old woman is brought into accident and emergency having been found unconscious by a friend in her room at the local university halls of residence. The friend reports that the patient has no chronic medical problems or previous serious illnesses but had been suffering from a cold the previous day. The patient is not known to be taking any medication, has no history of recreational drug use or alcohol abuse.

On examination, the patient is unconscious, with a Glasgow Coma Score of 3/15. Her temperature is 39.3°C. The pulse is 160/min and regular. The blood pressure is 75/45 mmHg. No focal neurological signs are present. There is a widespread purpuric, non-blanching rash. Vaginal examination is normal and in particular, no tampons are present. No needle track marks or signs of

trauma are found. The patient appears well nourished. There is no evidence of faecal or urinary incontinence.

The oxygen saturations on room air are 85 per cent, improving to only 90 per cent with high flow oxygen by mask. Urinary catheterization reveals a residual volume of just 20 mL. Urine output over the next 30 minutes is 5 mL. It is noted that the patient oozes blood persistently from the venepuncture wounds and develops a bruise at the site of the arterial blood gas (ABG) sampling despite reasonable pressure. Assorted emergency investigations are obtained.

Question 1

What process do the results of the full blood count and clotting tests indicate and what is its basic mechanism?

Answer 1

The clotting analysis exhibits prolongation of the international normalized ratio (INR), activated partial thromboplastin time ratio (APTTR) and thrombin time

Investigations

Arterial blood gases (obtained on room air)

pH	7.12	(7.35–7.45)
pO$_2$	6.9 kPa	(11.2–12.6 kPa)
pCO$_2$	6.4 kPa	(4.7–6.0 kPa)
HCO$_3^-$	14 mmol/L	(19–24 mmol/L)

Full blood count

Hb (female)	9.2 g/dL	(11.5–15.5 g/dL)
WCC	24 × 10^9/L	(4–11 × 10^9/L)
Neutrophils	21 × 10^9/L	
Platelets	33 × 10^9/L	(150–450 × 10^9/L)
MCV	81 fL	(75–95 fL)
MHC	31.3 pg	(28–33 pg)
MCHC	34.9 g/dL	(32–36 g/dL)

Clotting

INR	4.2	(0.9–1.1)
APTTR	3.4	(0.9–1.1)
TT	19 s	(14–16 s)
Fibrin degradation products	35 mg/mL	(<10 mg/mL)

Biochemistry

Na$^+$	137 mmol/L	(135–145 mmol/L)
K$^+$	5.6 mmol/L	(3.5–5 mmol/L)
Urea	10.4 mmol/L	(2.5–6.7 mmol/L)
Creatinine	250 μmol/L	(70–170 μmol/L)
Glucose	3.9 mmol/L	(3.5–5.5 mmol/L)

Chest X-ray	See Figure 45.1

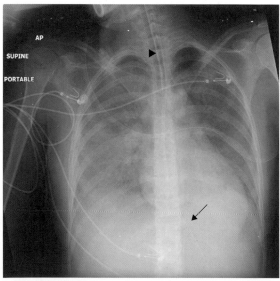

Figure 45.1 Typical portable ICU chest X-ray in a young patient with acute respiratory distress syndrome (ARDS) showing an endotracheal tube in the distal trachea (arrow head), a nasogastric tube with the tip placed in the stomach (arrow) and widespread 'airspace shadowing' or 'consolidation'. These ill-defined areas of opacity develop as fluid, pus (pneumonia), blood (Goodpasture's syndrome) or tumour (bronchioloalveolar carcinoma) fill the alveoli.

(TT), denoting a bleeding disorder that affects the whole of the coagulation cascade.

The elevated fibrin degradation products indicate widespread activation of the coagulation system in that they demonstrate that there has been a significant increase in the quantity of fibrinogen that has been activated and converted to fibrin, then degraded by fibrinolytic processes.

The full blood count reveals thrombocytopenia, implying that the platelet component of the clotting system is also deficient.

Further evidence of deranged clotting is present in the form of the patient's failure to clot at her venepuncture and ABG wounds.

The combination of widespread prolongation of clotting assays, thrombocytopenia and raised FDPs indicates disseminated intravascular coagulation (DIC).

DIC is a condition in which there is an aberrant, generalized activation of the clotting and fibrinolytic systems on a systemic scale, usually at the level of small blood vessels. Small microthrombi are formed and are broken down by the fibrinolytic system throughout the circulation. The process occurs on a sufficient level to deplete the reserves of the coagulation and/or fibrinolytic systems. Typically, the coagulation system succumbs to failure first, resulting in an overall bleeding disorder.

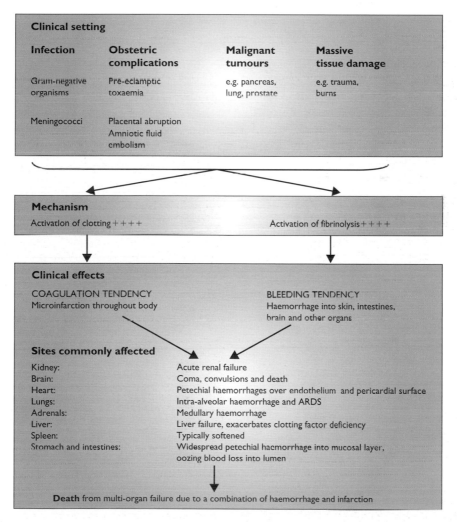

Figure 45.2 Disseminated intravascular coagulation (DIC): clinical settings and effects.

DIC has many causes which share the property of being forms of a severe, systemic insult.

Question 2

What does the information indicate about the patient's renal function and what is the likely cause?

Answer 2

The patient has acute renal failure. The low volume of urine in the bladder, given the lack of evidence to suggest that the patient had recently emptied her bladder, is the first indication of a low urine output. The formal measurement confirms this. As a general rule, the minimum acceptable urine output for an adult is 30–35 mL/hour. This may be refined to 0.5 mL/kg/hour, which is a useful guide for patients whose weight is significantly different from the 70 kg standard model.

The hyperkalaemia, elevated urea and creatinine are biochemical features of acute renal failure and reflect the failure of the kidney to excrete these substances adequately from the blood.

The cause of the renal failure is inadequate renal perfusion, secondary to marked hypotension. This is also known as prerenal acute renal failure. In the absence of an adequate blood flow and perfusion pressure, glomerular filtration fails. The low blood flow is also harmful to the tubular epithelium and thus a previously normal kidney is unable to function.

Question 3

What process has occurred in the lungs and what basic mechanism underlies it?

Answer 3

The blood gases show hypoxia, hypercapnia and an acidosis. This is type II respiratory failure.

Question 4

What derangement has occurred in the acid–base balance?

Answer 4

The acidosis is complex as the bicarbonate level is also low. In a pure respiratory acidosis, bicarbonate is normal or elevated, the latter occurring due to compensatory retention of bicarbonate by the kidney. However, in either a pure metabolic acidosis or a mixed metabolic and respiratory acidosis, bicarbonate levels are reduced as they are consumed by the excess hydrogen ions of the acid. In this case, the patient has a mixed respiratory and metabolic acidosis.

The respiratory component of the acidosis is a consequence of the impaired gas transfer leading to retention of carbon dioxide. This patient has two reasons to have a metabolic acidosis. First, acute renal failure is accompanied by a metabolic acidosis because the kidney is the normal route for excreting hydrogen ions. Second, the patient's severe hypotension will lead to significant organ hypoperfusion and a switch to anaerobic metabolism, with an accumulation of lactic acid.

Question 5

What is the diagnosis and what process underlies the complications above, together with the hypotension?

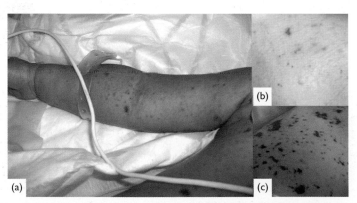

Figure 45.3 (a) Purpuric skin rash in a baby with meningococcal meningitis. (b) Early and (c) late meningococcal rash. The spots fail to blanch when viewed through a glass tumbler pressed against the skin. Most inflammatory rashes are caused by local vasodilatation but in disseminated intravascular coagulation (DIC)-associated rashes, such as that seen in meningococcal septicaemia, there is damage to capillary walls due to microthrombus formation, followed by haemorrhage into the skin. (Photographs reproduced with the kind permission of the Meningitis Research Foundation; www.meningitis.org.)

Answer 5

The clinical presentation is very characteristic of meningococcal septicaemia. The causative organism, *Neisseria meningitidis* (meningococcus), can also produce meningitis, but meningococcal septicaemia is often present in the absence of meningitis and vice versa.

Meningococcus wreaks much of its havoc in meningococcal septicaemia by the production of an endotoxin. The endotoxin damages endothelium, leading to increased permeability and thrombosis. Thus, the significant quantities of endotoxin that are spread throughout the vasculature have a route for triggering widespread foci of coagulation and initiating DIC.

Endotoxin also stimulates the production of large quantities of assorted cytokines by macrophages, including interkeukin 1 (IL-1), IL-6 and tumour necrosis factor (TNF). Considerable activation of complement also occurs and further drives an acute inflammatory response, thereby contributing to vasodilatation and

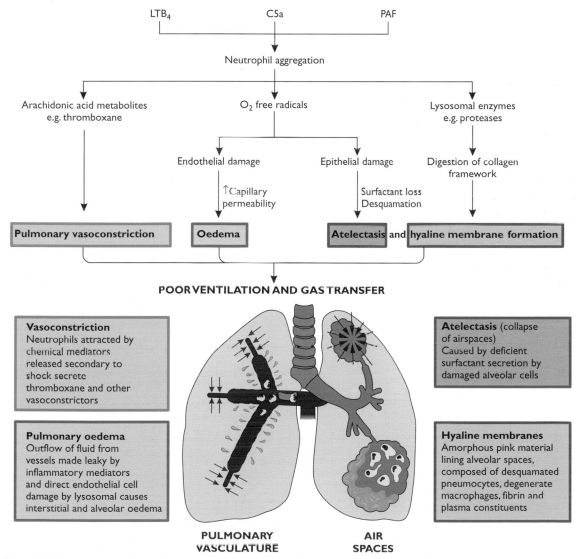

Figure 45.4 Pathogenesis of adult respiratory distress syndrome (ARDS). An initiating event causes shock. Acute inflammatory mediators damage vascular endothelium, the alveolar walls and lining epithelium and cause pulmonary vasoconstriction, oedema, collapse and the formation of membranes over the alveolar surface.

hypotension. TNF stimulates endothelial cells to produce nitric oxide. Nitric oxide is a powerful physiological vasodilator that is important in normal vascular regulation. If nitric oxide levels are inappropriately elevated throughout the vasculature, as can occur if driven by meningococcal endotoxin, hypotension and shock result. Nitric oxide-induced shock and hypotension are especially difficult to treat because the nitric oxide acts directly at the final step of the vasodilator pathway. Inhibitors of vasodilatation are generally unsuccessful because they interrupt the vasodilator pathway before nitric oxide has become involved. Instead, pressor agents are needed to drive the vasoconstrictor mechanisms.

Inhibitors of nitric oxide synthetase are in development. Caution will be necessary because nitric oxide is important in cerebral neurotransmission and cerebral blood flow autoregulation and disturbing these processes in a brain already suffering from the effects of septicaemic shock is not ideal. However, isoforms of the enzyme exist and may permit organ specificity.

Question 6

Why was specific reference made to the absence of a tampon?

Answer 6

Retained tampons can act as a focus for *Staphylococcus aureus* which then secretes an endotoxin that can cause the serious toxic shock syndrome.

SUMMARY

Although this case may seem to have many complex, independent elements, they all originate from the basic process of infection and the production of a toxin by the organism. The toxin has systemic access and operates at a systemic level. By inducing an inappropriately targeted, excessive, acute inflammatory response, the endotoxin induces profound vasodilatation and shock. As is typical of these processes, acute renal failure and acute respiratory distress syndrome (ARDS) result. DIC is a well-known companion to shock and endotoxin-mediated diseases and also supervenes.

Knowledge of the underlying mechanism shows that treatment should be aimed at removing the cause, which is the presence of the endotoxin that is itself secondary to the meningococcal septicaemia. Appropriate antibiotics are required to address this. Supportive care is also essential to counter the established effects of the endotoxin. This can be challenging but understanding how the organs are damaged and why they are failing permits optimal corrective measures to be taken.

A 59-year-old man presents to his GP with a one-month history of swelling of his ankles, urinary frequency and polydipsia. Further questioning also elicits a history of a reduced libido and shortness of breath on moderate exertion where this had not previously been a problem.

On examination, the patient seems to have a greyish tinge to his skin, although does not appear anaemic or cyanosed. There is mild pitting oedema of the ankles. The pulse is 88 beats per minute and irregularly irregular. The blood pressure is 135/84 mmHg. The jugular venous pressure (JVP) is not raised. The apex beat shows mild lateral displacement, but is normal in quality. No heaves or thrills are present. The first and second heart sound are normal and there are no murmurs or added sounds.

Examination of the lungs reveals bilateral basal crackles, but is otherwise normal. Abdominal examination is unremarkable. Examination of the external genitalia reveals testes that seem to show a mild degree of atrophy. No scrotal masses are present. Neurological examination is unremarkable.

The GP orders a variety of blood tests.

Investigations

Full blood count	Normal
Urea and electrolytes	Normal
Bilirubin	16 µg/L
GGT	134 IU/L
ALT	79 IU/L
Alk phos	90 IU/L
Albumin	37 g/L
Glucose	8 mmol/L (fasting venous)

A chest X-ray reveals a limited degree of upper lobe blood diversion and a mild increase in the width of the cardiac silhouette.

Question 1

What rhythm would the ECG be expected to demonstrate?

Answer 1

Atrial fibrillation. The irregularly irregular pulse is typical. In the case of this patient, no additional abnormalities were present.

Question 2

What additional cardiac process is occurring?

Answer 2

Cardiac failure of a relatively mild degree. The patient has exertional dyspnoea, coupled with peripheral oedema and evidence of pulmonary oedema on clinical examination and chest X-ray. Given that the patient's pulse rate is in the normal range, the atrial fibrillation alone may well not be sufficient to explain the impaired cardiac function.

Question 3

What endocrine abnormality(ies) does this patient have?

Answer 3

The elevated fasting blood glucose indicates diabetes mellitus. This would also explain the polyuria and polydipsia due to an osmotic diuresis induced by glycosuria.

There is also likely to be an element of hypogonadism. There has been a change in the patient's libido and there seems to be some degree of testicular atrophy. Further investigation would reveal that the patient had a low blood follicle-stimulating hormone (FSH), luteinizing hormone (LH) and testosterone.

Question 4

What is the diagnosis?

Answer 4

The patient has haemochromatosis. He has abnormal liver function tests, cardiac disease, diabetes mellitus, pituitary disease (hypogonadism secondary to decreased levels of the FSH and LH from the pituitary) and characteristic skin pigmentation changes.

Question 5

What is haemochromatosis?

Answer 5

Haemochromatosis is an autosomal recessive disease in which there is an abnormal increase in iron absorption from the gut.

Question 6

How could the diagnosis be confirmed?

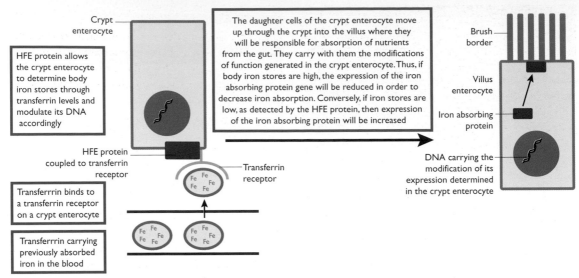

Crypt enterocyte

HFE protein allows the crypt enterocyte to determine body iron stores through transferrin levels and modulate its DNA accordingly

The daughter cells of the crypt enterocyte move up through the crypt into the villus where they will be responsible for absorption of nutrients from the gut. They carry with them the modifications of function generated in the crypt enterocyte. Thus, if body iron stores are high, the expression of the iron absorbing protein gene will be reduced in order to decrease iron absorption. Conversely, if iron stores are low, as detected by the HFE protein, then expression of the iron absorbing protein will be increased

Brush border

Villus enterocyte

Iron absorbing protein

HFE protein coupled to transferrin receptor

Transferrin receptor

DNA carrying the modification of its expression determined in the crypt enterocyte

Transferrrin binds to a transferrin receptor on a crypt enterocyte

Transferrrin carrying previously absorbed iron in the blood

Figure 46.1 Control of absorption of iron from the gut.

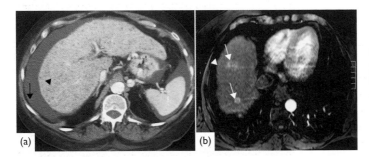

(a)   (b)

Figure 46.2 (a) Axial CT in a haemochromatosis patient with nodular cirrhosis (arrow head) with multiple small nodules scattered through the liver and ascites (thin arrow). (b) Axial T2 MRI of the liver showing two hepatocellular carcinomas (thin arrows) in a haemochromatosis liver – a complication of cirrhosis. Note the nodular margin of the liver (arrow head) a feature of cirrhosis.

Answer 6

Genetic studies can be performed and are the most useful, but measurement of iron transport and storage levels in the blood is also helpful and quicker. Liver biopsy can reveal the presence of excess iron, as well as assessing other histological parameters and permitting measurement of the total iron content.

The gene for haemochromatosis is located on chromosome 6p21.3, although alternative loci have been described for variants of the disease. The protein is called HFE. There is a linkage with the HLA types A3 and B14.

excess iron is present in the free form. Free iron is actually toxic and causes damage because it induces the generation of free radicals. The tissue damages triggers a chronic inflammatory response that includes fibrosis.

Different organs will show different degrees of susceptibility to haemochromatosis, due in part to their roles in normal iron metabolism. As the body's main metabolic centre and iron reservoir, the liver is especially vulnerable. However, the heart, pancreas, skin and pituitary are also at particular risk. Iron deposition and the ensuing chronic inflammation and fibrosis damage these organs, leading to impaired organ function.

Question 7

How does haemochromatosis cause disease?

Answer 7

The elevated absorption of iron from the gut overwhelms the body's storage capacity for iron. This means that the

Question 8

What patterns of change can occur in the liver?

Answer 8

The liver has surprisingly few basic patterns of response to injury, although these are often coloured by assorted

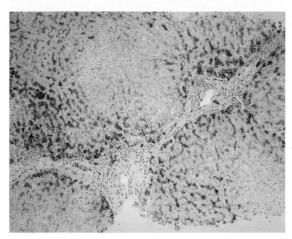

Figure 46.3 Cirrhotic liver showing bright blue positivity with Perl's stain for haemosiderin. This is grade 4 (of 4) haemosiderosis. Most of the iron is within liver parenchymal cells, suggesting a genetic aetiology, rather than in Kupffer cells, where surplus dietary iron or transfusional iron overload is first apparent.

nuances for specific diseases. In haemochromatosis, the liver changes at presentation tend to fall in the spectrum of chronic hepatitis, active chronic hepatitis, cirrhosis and hepatocellular carcinoma. As a general rule, anything that causes active chronic hepatitis can cause cirrhosis and anything that can cause cirrhosis can cause hepatocellular carcinoma, but the tendency with which cirrhosis can lead to hepatocellular carcinoma does vary.

Question 9

Is liver biopsy important if the diagnosis has already been made?

Answer 9

Even if the diagnosis has been confirmed through other means, liver biopsy remains important in haemochromatosis in order to evaluate the extent of the liver damage. The distinction between fibrosis without cirrhosis and cirrhosis is important.

Question 10

Given that haemochromatosis is a disease of iron overload, what treatment would seem appropriate?

Answer 10

It is not currently possible to correct the abnormality in the bowel that causes the increased absorption of iron. However, it is possible to remove the excess iron. Regular venesection is a simple mechanism for extracting iron from the body and avoids the use of chelating agents and their attendant side-effects. Venesection can produce quite marked improvements in organ function, but cannot reverse established cirrhosis.

Question 11

Why do women who have haemochromatosis tend to present later than men?

Answer 11

Women of reproductive age have natural blood loss in the form of menstruation. This can be sufficient to hold the disease at bay until after the menopause.

Gavin Solaros is a 33-year-old futures trader in the City of London. The element of risk appeals to him and he is well paid for his nerve and success. His lifestyle is lavish. Gourmet feasts are accompanied by the finest wines and spirits. One evening, Gavin polishes off a bottle of claret with a delicious plate of roast guinea fowl. Suddenly he is seized by a searing pain in his epigastrium, which radiates through to his back. He is nauseated and vomits – the great wine is wasted! He doubles up but no change of position relieves the agony.

Gavin summons his GP, who notes that the abdomen is extremely tender, with peritonism. Bowel sounds are absent. He has a pyrexia of 38.3°C, blood pressure of 100/60 mmHg and tachycardia of 118 beats per minute, sinus rhythm. Gavin is urgently admitted to hospital.

Question 1

List and comment on your differential diagnosis.

Answer 1

- Perforated duodenal or gastric peptic ulcer: abdominal X-ray would show gas under the diaphragm if the free wall is perforated; perforation into the pancreas would cause a moderate rise in pancreatic amylase and back pain.
- Acute pancreatitis: he is rather young. 80–95 per cent of cases have a history of gallstones or alcohol abuse. Look for pyrexia, tachycardia, mild jaundice, bleeding into flank or around umbilicus. Serum amylase >1000 IU/L is diagnostic.
- Acute appendicitis: unusual symptoms and signs unless appendix is long and retrocaecal.
- Biliary colic, acute cholecystitis: look for jaundice, dark urine. Rather young. Pain is usually colicky. May precede pancreatitis.
- Ureteric colic: usually a griping pain, possibly accompanied by loin pain on affected side if pyelonephritis is present, may have haematuria or dysuria.
- Meckel's diverticulitis with perforation – rare! Meckel's diverticulum occurs in 2 per cent of the population, but few contain ectopic pancreatic or gastric mucosa which increase the risk of perforation.
- Intestinal obstruction by torsion, intussusception, Crohn's stricture, infarction: pain would not usually radiate to the back.

- At this age, diverticulitis, carcinomatous obstruction or perforation or abdominal aortic aneurysm are unlikely.

In hospital, Gavin's blood and urine are tested. An abdominal ultrasound and CT scan show a few small gallstones in the gallbladder, but no stone obstructs the common bile duct (CBD). The pancreas is swollen. He settles on non-morphine-derived painkillers and intravenous fluids.

The test results return.

Investigations

Hb	11.3 g/dL
WCC	13.5×10^9/dL
Platelets	200×10^{12}/dL
Urea	High normal
Creatinine	High normal
Calcium	Low normal
Glucose	Slight increase
Blood gases	Normal
	Slight acidosis
Amylase	1340 IU/L

A diagnosis of acute pancreatitis is made. He is reassured that his attack could have been far worse.

Question 2

What is the mechanism underlying acute pancreatitis? What are the long-term complications?

Answer 2

In 60 per cent of cases, it is due to gallstone obstruction of the CBD and pancreatic duct, with bile reflux into the pancreatic duct.

Twenty per cent of cases are due to alcohol, possibly a directly toxic effect. Alcohol causes extremely viscid mucous secretions which can result in protein plugs that obstruct small and large pancreatic ducts.

Obstruction causes inflammation and autodigestion of the pancreas by its wide range of enzymes. Lipases digest adjacent fat, proteases the pancreas itself and elastases demolish the walls of blood vessels. Severe bleeding into the pancreas and retroperitoneal tissues can result and this may track into the flanks and around the umbilicus to cause bruising (Cullen's and Grey–Turner's signs, respectively).

Acute pancreatitis is life-threatening. Some patients spend months in intensive care.

Adverse features (Ranson's criteria) are:

- very high white cell count
- low haemoglobin
- raised urea
- raised liver enzymes
- inflammatory ascites
- raised glucose
- metabolic acidosis
- low blood pO_2 levels
- age more than 55 years

Long-term complications include:

- pancreatic pseudocyst: fluid and blood accumulate in the destroyed pancreatic tissue.
- chronic pancreatitis: acute does not necessarily precede chronic pancreatitis.
- diabetes mellitus due to damage to the islets of Langerhans.

Gavin returns to work, shaken, 12 weeks later. He has been advised to avoid alcohol.

Unusually, he finds himself anxious. He finds that alcohol improves his performance. He starts taking a hip flask containing vodka to work. His trading decisions are erratic. He has regular check-ups with his GP, but resents the constant questioning about his alcohol intake. His colleagues comment that he has become withdrawn. Sometimes his breath smells of alcohol mid-morning. He is defensive and aggressive when questioned, and then suddenly dissolves into tears. Embarrassed, they shuffle him out of the building and home in a taxi before their employers see him.

His GP tells him that he is depressed, which may be linked to his continued alcohol consumption, and adds, 'Can I ask you some questions, called a CAGE test?'

'Just give me some pills and leave me alone,' snarls Gavin rudely. The GP prescribes antidepressants. Once he has gone, Gavin turns once more to his cellar and comforts himself with a deliciously crisp bottle of Pouilly Fumé with … no, he doesn't feel like eating. He rounds off his evening with a glass of vintage port.

Question 3

What psychiatric manifestations of alcohol dependence are seen in Gavin? What is the CAGE test, and does he score positively?

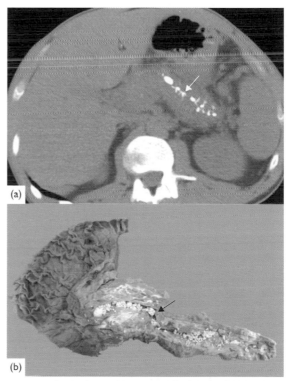

Figure 47.2 (a) Chronic alcohol-related pancreatitis with calcifications in the pancreatic duct (arrow). (b) The appearances are mirrored in this pathological specimen showing the pancreas and duodenum.

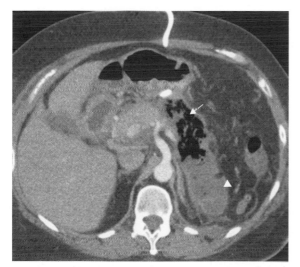

Figure 47.1 CT of acute pancreatitis with the tail of the pancreas replaced by fluid (arrow head) pancreatic necrosis and gas in a pancreatic abscess (thin arrow).

Answer 3

- Inability to concentrate
- Depression
- Emotional lability.

The CAGE test is a four-question test developed by Dr John Ewing:

- Have you ever felt you should cut down on your alcohol intake?
- Have you been annoyed by someone criticizing your alcohol intake?
- Have you ever felt guilty about your drinking?
- Have you ever had to take a drink first thing in the morning ('eye-opener') to recover from drinking the night before or to steady your nerves?

Gavin has another bout of severe abdominal pain with fever. Back in hospital, the CT scan shows calcified areas in his pancreas. He is diagnosed with chronic pancreatitis, treated with analgesics and has his fluid balance restored. After four weeks he is discharged and advised to avoid alcohol at all costs.

Question 4

Is chronic pancreatitis related to alcohol?

Answer 4

Yes, alcohol is the main association, and gallstones are also implicated in recurrent acute pancreatitis.

When Gavin finally returns to work, he is summoned to the chief executive's office. Serious trading misdemeanours have been identified. With a shock Gavin recalled that he had meant to cover up some major losses about three months ago. He is sacked.

After a year Gavin can no longer meet his mortgage repayments and his penthouse suite is repossessed. He moves to a small flat in the suburbs. He cannot get another city job and has brief stints at jobs with easy access to alcohol, losing each within weeks for unreliability.

Another bout of chronic pancreatitis occurs about three years after the first episode, this time taking many weeks to recover. Gavin is now approaching 40 and is greying and haggard, with early clawing of his hands (Dupuytren's contractures). He is now homeless. He begs for money and buys beer or spirits. He suffers painful attacks of gout in his fingers and his right big toe.

Question 5

What is gout and why are alcohol drinkers at increased risk?

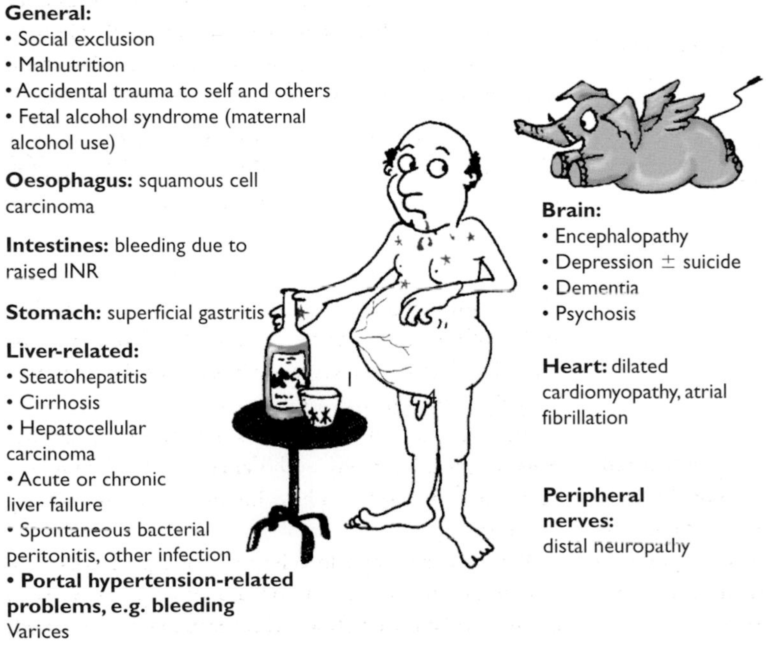

General:
- Social exclusion
- Malnutrition
- Accidental trauma to self and others
- Fetal alcohol syndrome (maternal alcohol use)

Oesophagus: squamous cell carcinoma

Intestines: bleeding due to raised INR

Stomach: superficial gastritis

Liver-related:
- Steatohepatitis
- Cirrhosis
- Hepatocellular carcinoma
- Acute or chronic liver failure
- Spontaneous bacterial peritonitis, other infection
- **Portal hypertension-related problems, e.g. bleeding** Varices

Brain:
- Encephalopathy
- Depression ± suicide
- Dementia
- Psychosis

Heart: dilated cardiomyopathy, atrial fibrillation

Peripheral nerves: distal neuropathy

Figure 47.3 The diagram reinforces the fact that alcohol does not only damage the liver. It is likely that alcohol may play a less direct role in other diseases.

Answer 5

Uric acid is a product of purine metabolism. High uric acid levels in the blood, from over-ingestion, over-production or reduced excretion of uric acid, cause deposition of monosodium urate crystals in joints, typically the big toe. Gouty joints are exquisitely painful and are hot, red and very swollen. Attacks last about 2–3 days.

Beer and some spirits contain high levels of purines, as do bacon, beans, liver and shellfish. Alcohol stimulates diuresis, raising the blood uric acid concentration. Male sex is important and genetic factors may be contributory.

Gavin throws himself under a bus, but only breaks his right humerus. He is admitted to hospital once more. The bones will not unite. 'You are so malnourished,' a kindly night nurse explains to him. 'You must try to eat properly. We are giving you extra vitamins.'

Question 6

What can cause malnutrition in chronic alcoholics?

Answer 6

- Chronic pancreatitis: pancreatic acinar destruction and fibrous replacement can cause pancreatic enzyme deficiency and malabsorption.
- Alcoholics often neglect food because the alcohol can be metabolized to give energy. Vitamin deficiencies develop, particularly the water-soluble B vitamins, which are poorly stored in the body. Thiamine (vitamin B_1) deficiency is most common.
- Money is spent on alcohol rather than food. Loss of employment exacerbates this element.

Question 7

Which nutrients are most important in bone healing?

Answer 7

- Vitamin C
- Zinc
- Protein
- Oxygen
- Vitamin D and calcium.

Gavin becomes breathless during his stay in hospital. The junior doctor has been reading about alcohol-related conditions and considers a diagnosis of alcoholic cardiomyopathy. Then Gavin coughs up purulent sputum – he has developed a chest infection with *Pseudomonas aeruginosa*, resistant to all first-line antibiotics.

Question 8

What is the significance of this infection?

Answer 8

Pseudomonas aeruginosa is a typical example of a hospital-acquired infection, and is often resistant to the standard first-line antibiotics for chest infections. Alcoholics are particularly susceptible to infection by encapsulated bacteria.

Question 9

Does alcohol cause a cardiomyopathy?

Answer 9

There are three main types of cardiomyopathy – hypertrophic, dilated and restrictive. Alcohol is one of several causes of dilated cardiomyopathy.

At last Gavin is told he can go home. Nobody checks that he has a home to go to.

He wanders the streets. A policeman takes him to a night shelter, where he is fed and housed. Gavin has difficulty with simple physical tasks like doing up buttons. After a few years he becomes very confused and forgetful and invents stories to explain away the gaps in his memory.

One day, over the course of a few hours, he begins to stagger, with eyes rolling – he seems drunk. The experienced hostel manager recognizes Wernicke–Korsakoff's type dementia. He takes Gavin to hospital. There is little that the psychiatric department can offer him, other than vitamin B injections.

Question 10

Can alcohol cause the symptoms displayed by Gavin?

Answer 10

Gavin's fumbling indicates a sensorimotor neuropathy, which often affects the feet and hands. Alcohol may be directly toxic or act via vitamin deficiencies (particularly B_{12}, thiamine and vitamin E).

Malnutrition of B vitamins (especially thiamine) causes cortical atrophy with damage to the hypothalamus and mamillary bodies, important for processing memories.

Wernicke's encephalopathy comprises paralysis of eye muscles, nystagmus, confusion and major problems with balance and co-ordination, with a strikingly wide-based, irregular and staggering gait. Patients are often misdiagnosed as being drunk, so delaying treatment. Wernicke's encephalopathy may rapidly progress to coma and death if vitamin B_1 is not infused immediately – the brain damage already incurred cannot be repaired. Twenty per cent of patients with Wernicke's encephalopathy die; 85 per cent of Wernicke's encephalopathy survivors will develop Korsakoff's psychosis (amnesic-confabulatory syndrome), caused by thiamine deficiency. Patients fill the gaps in their memories by inventing stories. They often show personality alterations.

One winter's night, Gavin falls asleep on an icy bench outside the city firm where he once was a rising star. He never awakens.

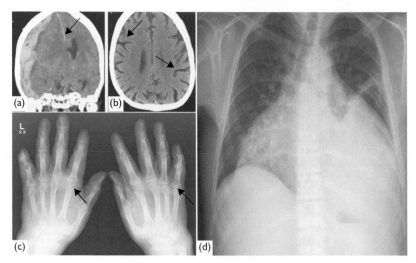

Figure 47.4 (a) Coronal CT in a patient with a head injury after a drinking binge showing a large subdural haematoma (arrowhead) associated with mass effect, midline shift and subfalcine herniation (arrow). (b) Cerebral atrophy in a 35-year-old man with chronic alcohol abuse. Note the depth and prominence of the cerebral sulci (arrow). (c) Hand X-rays of a patient with gout with erosive changes in the joints (arrows), joint deformities and preservation of bone density. (d) Chest X-ray showing congestive cardiomyopathy in a 50-year-old male patient with chronic alcohol abuse . Note the massive heart and the plethoric lungs.

CASE 48

CERTIFYING THE CAUSE OF DEATH

This book, *Pathology in Clinical Practice*, would not be complete without some practice in deciding how to certify the cause of death. It is the duty of doctors to provide the 'Medical Certificate of Cause of Death' to bereaved relatives and to know when to refer cases to the coroner, so let us use some of the scenarios in the book to illustrate the key points.

Question 1

Look back at Case 1, Intermittent chest pain (p.2) and imagine that the man progresses to suffer from unstable angina, is seen regularly by his doctor and then suddenly collapses and dies while watching a crucial cup match at his local football club. There are no suspicious circumstances. What would you write as cause of death on the death certificate? A copy of the certificates used in the UK is shown as Figure 48.1. This is closely similar to those of other countries, but some allow for four lines of sequential conditions under I.

Answer 1

He has a clearly diagnosed condition, unstable angina, that can result in sudden death and no reasons to suspect any other cause so the death certificate would show:

I (a) Acute myocardial ischaemia
  (b) Coronary artery atheroma

Question 2

What are death certificates used for?

Answer 2

The death certificate is needed by the relatives so that they can register the death. What is written as the cause of death and how the death is explained to them by the healthcare professionals involved can help them come to terms with the loss, so it is important to take time to do this well. The data are recorded by the General

BIRTHS AND DEATHS REGISTRATION ACT 1953
(Form prescribed by Registration of Births and Deaths Regulations 1987)

Registrar to enter No. of Death Entry

MEDICAL CERTIFICATE OF CAUSE OF DEATH
For use only by a Registered Medical Practitioner WHO HAS BEEN IN ATTENDANCE during the deceased s last illness, and to be delivered by him forthwith to the Registrar of Births and Deaths.

Name of deceased ....
Date of death as stated to me .... day of .... Age as stated to me ....
Place of death ....
Last seen alive by me .... day of ....

1 The certified cause of death takes account of information obtained from post-mortem.
2 Information from post-mortem may be available later
3 Post mortem not being held.
4 I have reported this death to the Coroner for further action. *(See overleaf)*

Please ring appropriate digit(s) and letter

a Seen after death by me.
b Seen after death by another medical practitioner but not by me
c Not seen after death by a medical practitioner.

SPECIMEN

CAUSE OF DEATH
The condition thought to be the Underlying Cause of Death should appear in the lowest completed line of Part I.

I (a) Disease or condition directly leading to death† ....
(b) Other disease or condition, if any, leading to: I(a) ....
(c) Other disease or condition, if any, leading to: I(b) ....

II Other significant conditions **CONTRIBUTING TO THE DEATH** but not related to the disease or condition causing it ....

These particulars not to be entered in death register
Approximate interval between onset and death

The death might have been due to or contributed to by the employment followed at some time by the deceased ☐ Please tick where applicable

This does not mean the mode of dying, such as heart failure, asphyxia, asthenia, etc: it means the disease, injury, or complication which caused death.

I hereby certify that I was in medical attendance during the above named deceased s last illness, and that the particulars and cause of death above written are true to the best of my knowledge and belief.

Signature .... Qualifications as registered by General Medical Council ....
Residence .... Date ....

For deaths in hospital: Please give the name of the consultant responsible for the above- named as a patient ....

Figure 48.1 A specimen copy of the death certificate that is completed by doctors in England and Wales.

Register Office (in England and Wales), collated and analysed by the Office of National Statistics and used by researchers and health planners to assess health needs and the impact of interventions.

Question 3

Let's try another case. Look back at Case 12, Permanent neurological signs (p. 44) and imagine that this woman did not return home, because she was unable to care for herself, and was looked after in a nursing home. Here she became depressed, ate little and rarely moved out of bed. She developed a productive cough but had indicated in her Advance Decision to Refuse Treatment (ADRT) that she did not want to receive antibiotics. She died 48 hours later. Her notes indicate that she had a malignant breast lump removed three years ago and was not thought to have any recurrence. What would you write on her death certificate?

Answer 3

I (a) Bronchopneumonia
   (b) Left cerebral infarction
   (c) Cerebrovascular disease
II Breast cancer

The sequence of events here is that the final cause of death is her chest infection, which translates into medical terminology as bronchopneumonia. That is unlikely to have killed her if she had not already had a 'stroke'. Her 'stroke' was an ischaemic one (rather than a haemorrhagic one) and would have resulted in necrosis of cerebral tissue (cerebral infarction) with the underlying cause being narrowed and atheromatous arteries (cerebrovascular disease).

Section II of the cause of death is for 'Other significant conditions contributing to the death but not related to the disease or condition causing it'. This can be a very tricky decision. Has the breast cancer actually contributed to the death? Might she have been less depressed and more keen to accept antibiotics if she had not already had a malignant tumour and possibly feared that it might recur or spread? You have to use your judgement, but it is generally acceptable to indicate serious conditions under II so that the epidemiologists can use it if they wish.

Question 4

How is the death certificate data collated and analysed?

Answer 4

The World Health Organization co-ordinates the production of coding systems suitable for use across the world that allow comparisons to be made over time and between different countries. The relevant one for death certificates is the *International Statistical Classification of*

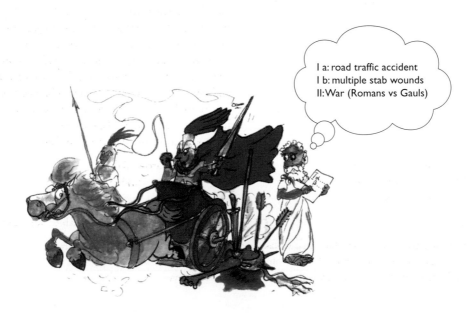

I a: road traffic accident
I b: multiple stab wounds
II: War (Romans vs Gauls)

Figure 48.2 Be as precise as possible in selecting the actual cause of death for section I, and include contributing factors in section II.

Diseases and Related Health Problems, 10th revision known affectionately as 'ICD-10'. The diagnoses reported on adult death certificates are coded automatically using software, a complex set of rules and the codes contained in the three volumes of ICD-10. It is the *underlying cause of death* that is coded and this should occupy the lowest completed line of part I. If you have difficulty organizing the sequence of events in part I, look at the figures you have put in the 'approximate interval between onset and death' box. The 'underlying cause' should have the longest duration.

Question 5

By now you will have appreciated that understanding the basic mechanisms of disease is the key to putting together the sequence of events that led to death, so let us just reinforce that with three more cases that you have already encountered.

1. Case 3, Difficulty in passing urine (p. 9). Imagine that this man has lived another decade but has become increasingly confused and is brought to accident and emergency with severe cardiac failure and is found to have pericarditis, and markedly raised blood urea and abnormal electrolytes. He dies the following morning. What do you put as the cause of death?

2. Case 31, Investigation after death (p. 118). This case has had an autopsy and you need to indicate in the upper part of the certificate whether you have taken the autopsy information into account. If not, you need to keep notes of the autopsy outcome so that you can provide further information when contacted. What are you going to give as the cause of death after attending the autopsy?

3. Case 23, Complex blood results (p. 90). This man with myeloma is treated for the next three years with intermittent chemotherapy to reduce the malignant plasma cell load. At the age of 72 years he has become a little breathless with features of mild heart failure and then drops dead half way round his favourite golf course. How do you complete the death certificate?

Answer 5a

He is known to have had benign prostatic hyperplasia a decade ago and this is a condition which is slowly progressive so he is likely to have developed increasing

urethral obstruction. That could have caused repeated infective episodes and/or raised back pressure affecting both kidneys. This would be supported by the finding of abnormal blood urea and electrolytes which occurs in chronic renal failure. His final cause of death will be acute cardiac failure, which can involve any combination of the cardiovascular consequences of acute or chronic renal failure (i.e. retention of fluid, hypertension, arrythmias due to raised potassium, pericarditis due to uraemia). So the death certificate would show:

I (a) Acute cardiac failure
  (b) chronic renal failure
  (c) benign prostatic hyperplasia.

Answer 5b

The autopsy has demonstrated metastases in most vital organs but no acute terminal event (such as massive haemorrhage from the ulcerated gut lesions). Thus, it is acceptable to put:

I (a) Multi-organ failure
  (b) multiple metastases
  (c) malignant melanoma.

Answer 5c

If you are his GP treating his mild heart failure and expected to complete the death certificate it would be worth checking with the specialist looking after his myeloma whether there was any suggestion of cardiac amyloid and what his ECGs had looked like. This is a case where an autopsy might provide useful information about the effectiveness of his myeloma treatment and precise cause of his cardiac problems; but since this is natural death with a variety of possible causes, it does not require referral to the coroner.

A possible cause of death would be:

I (a) Acute cardiac failure
  (b) cardiac amyloid
  (c) myeloma.

Without an autopsy, an acceptable alternative could be:

I (a) Acute myocardial ischaemia
  (b) atherosclerosis
II Myeloma.

Certifying the cause of death is closely similar in most countries around the world. The law will differ, however, on when you should *not* complete the death certificate but must refer the death for further investigation. This section explains the position for England and Wales at the time of publication. If you are practising in another country, make sure that you understand the local law.

Question 1

The doctor who has been in attendance during the deceased's last illness is required to provide a medical certificate of death if they are able to. What are the circumstances in which a doctor should *not* complete the death certificate?

Answer 1

You should not issue the certificate if you were not in attendance during the deceased's *last* illness. Refer it to the doctor who was.

You may complete the certificate if you are referring the case to the coroner, provided that you clearly indicate that you have referred it to the coroner for further action. Generally, though, it is better not to complete the certificate if you think it should be a coroner's case. It can cause confusion and distress to the relatives if they try to register the death.

Question 2

When should you refer cases to the coroner?

Answer 2

Currently there is a common law duty in England and Wales on all people to refer relevant cases to the coroner. The guidelines on what to refer are indicative rather than prescriptive and this is going to change with the introduction of legislation that will create a statutory duty on doctors and other public service personnel to report deaths to the coroner. The details are not finalized, but the list is likely to include:

- Deaths resulting from self-harm and neglect.
- Deaths resulting from neglect or abuse when there is an established duty of care by a public authority, other organizations and individuals.
- Deaths occurring during or shortly after a period of detention (e.g. in police custody, by military authorities or under the Mental Health Act).
- Death caused or contributed to by the police's conduct.

- Deaths related to employment.
- Death resulting from lack of care or appropriate treatment, defective treatment and adverse reaction to prescribed medicine.
- Death of a child ('where the death of that child was not anticipated as a significant possibility 24 hours before death').
- Deaths where a violent crime is suspected.
- Sudden and/or accidental death.
- A death that is the subject of significant concern or suspicion.
- Where the death has not been certified (because no doctor has attended the patient recently).
- A death that may have been caused or contributed to by a specified disease or condition. This is an innovation which, under new legislation, would involve the chief coroner specifying certain conditions as reportable. Possible examples are severe acute respiratory syndrome (SARS), tuberculosis, deep vein thrombosis associated with air travel, avian flu.
- Deaths associated with childbirth or termination of pregnancy.

For most doctors, that can be summarized as:

- unexpected
- unknown
- unnatural
- suspicious.

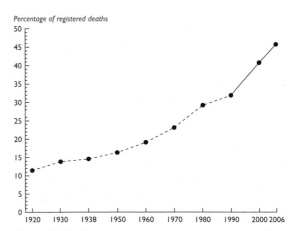

Figure 49.1 Deaths reported to coroners as a percentage of registered deaths, England and Wales. (Redrawn from data in Coroners' Annual Statistics 2006 available at www.dca.gov.uk/statistics/coroners.htm. Crown copyright material is reproduced with the permission of the Controller of HMSO and the Queen's Printer for Scotland.)

Question 3

Using that list as a guide, look back at Case 18, Tachycardia and tachypnoea (p.67) and decide whether you would refer to the coroner in each of the following scenarios:

(a) She is admitted to hospital, commences appropriate treatment but suffers a further massive pulmonary embolism, which kills her.

(b) Instead of calling the ambulance, she requests a GP home visit. Her GP knows that she suffers from asthma and is susceptible to chest infections and prescribes antibiotics and bed rest. She dies later that day.

(c) Instead of calling the ambulance, she takes some painkillers and decides to try to sleep off her jet lag. She doesn't wake up.

Answer 3a

There is no need to refer to the coroner unless, in the future, the chief coroner stipulates that transatlantic flight-related deaths should be referred. Pulmonary

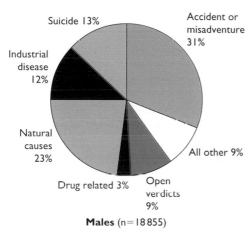

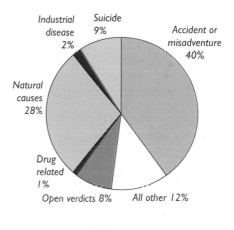

Figure 49.2 Verdicts returned at inquest by sex, England and Wales, 2006. (Redrawn from data in Coroners' Annual Statistics 2006 available at www.dca.gov.uk/statistics/coroners.htm. Crown copyright material is reproduced with the permission of the Controller of HMSO and the Queen's Printer for Scotland.)

embolism is a natural death, the diagnosis has been established and it is not suspicious. She has been correctly treated, however, bereaved relatives may question the care when faced with a sudden unexpected death and they may suggest referral. Then it would be wise to agree.

Answer 3b

It is the GP who is the doctor in attendance and he or she must refer to the coroner because the death is unexpected. Even if the GP believes that the cause of death is a chest infection, a healthy 51-year-old would not be expected to die suddenly.

Answer 3c

This must be referred to the coroner and those involved need to investigate the full range of possible causes, including the unnatural and suspicious ones.

This requires the coroner's officers to question the relatives and a pathologist to perform an autopsy. The information from these two sources is then discussed so that a certificate is issued or an inquest is held. In this case, the autopsy would show a natural cause of death (pulmonary embolism) and no inquest is required.

Question 4

From the previous case (Certifying the cause of death, p. 191) look again at Question 5a and decide whether it should be referred to the coroner.

Answer 4

The confused 82-year-old does not sound to have received adequate care over the last few months or years but it is difficult to judge without knowing more of his social history. If in doubt, phone the coroner's officer for advice. Ultimately it is your responsibility to decide whether to refer, but taking advice is prudent.

Question 5

You have signed the death certificate on one of your patients and the relatives are planning a cremation so you are asked to complete the cremation form. What is the crucial thing that you have to do before signing a cremation certificate that you do not have to do before signing a death certificate?

Answer 5

You *must* see the body. The death certificate requires you to indicate whether you have seen the deceased after death, whether another medical practitioner has or whether no practitioner has, but does not require you to see it. For a cremation form, you must personally see and examine the body. The nature of the examination is not specified and simple inspection is sufficient if the person is long dead and has been dealt with by funeral directors or other health professionals. If you are the first to see the body, it is wise to turn it over to spot the knife in the back.

CASE 50

Sarah McKenzie had not spent five years at medical school without learning to ignore the swarm of low-flying rumours that buzzed around as the misleading harbingers of the next exam to lurk on the horizon, but neither had she made the mistake of underestimating the resilience of medical students in garnering intelligence ahead of the latest confrontation between student and faculty. With her finals now upon her, she had every reason to believe that the talk of the pathology department unleashing a new, secret weapon was true. There was to be an additional paper and in the absence of facts, the students had started to speculate. Rather than waste valuable revision time trying to ascertain the future, Sarah endeavoured to devote her energy to learning about those subjects she knew from her training were relevant.

On the day of the first exam, one of Sarah's friends, Kelly, had, according to Kelly's own assessment, made an absolute mess of the pathology paper. Hours of attempts at reassurance had done little to ameliorate the situation and had predictably degenerated into a long and tearful discussion on the part of Kelly about what could come up in the infamous new extra paper, which would be upon them the following morning. By the time Kelly had been soothed by sympathetic listening and a revision session in which Sarah had tested her, from textbooks and lecture notes, on all manner of subjects, it was just after one in the morning before Sarah returned to her bed.

There had been occasions before when Sarah had turned over an exam paper and found that the first question centred on a topic with which she was not particularly comfortable, or was frankly unfamiliar to her. A couple of times she had experienced the first cold pangs of fear when the second question had also fallen outside the boundaries of her expectation, but as she made her way through the pages of the dreaded pathology paper, there was no familiar point of anchorage for her, no place at which she could set down her pen and begin the challenge from a secure base. The icy sensation that gripped her was much worse than a mere chill of alarm and she could see her aspirations for the future, for her career, crumbling into fine dust that would be blown away with her next breath. *Not one single disease did she recognize in the paper.*

Sarah looked around the examination hall, as candidates do when, in desperation, they try to seek some comfort in the fact that most of their colleagues are suffering similar difficulties. The confusion and distress on the faces of the rest of the candidates mirrored her own. As the final test, Sarah, moved her gaze to her friend Thomas, the person that the rest of the year would look to as the top of the class. Thomas's face bore what seemed to Sarah to be an incongruous smile, an expression that a chess player might adopt when he appreciates the ingenuity of an opponent's move, yet perceives in the same instance of this admiration that he can reply to it, defeat its cleverness and ultimately smash it from the board.

Sarah returned her attention to the paper. Other than Thomas, everybody had the same problem. She did not allow herself to be distracted by speculation as to whether or not the medical school would really be prepared to fail almost the entire year. Keeping calm and focusing on technique could yet go a long way.

Deciding to adopt a methodical approach, Sarah began with the first part of question 1 as it was at least something she could do, even if the reference to the condition of Jacobs–Tate syndrome in the preceding preamble suggested that much of the question would be beyond her, given that she had never heard of Jacobs–Tate syndrome.

'What is the GABA-A receptor?'

'The GABA-A receptor is a CNS neurotransmitter receptor for gamma-aminobutyric acid,' wrote Sarah. 'The binding of GABA opens a chloride channel, which has an inhibitory effect on the neurone.'

'What is the mechanism of action of benzodiazepines?'

Again, this was safe territory. Sarah liked pharmacology because it allowed her to correlate normal physiology and biochemistry with functional effects and rewarded the effort put in to learning those normal processes.

'Benzodiazepines bind to the GABA-A receptor and allosterically modify it so that its frequency of opening is increased when GABA binds. This increases the effect of GABA on the receptor.'

At least Sarah had a couple of marks to her name now, although she had no idea how talk of the GABA-A receptor related to the main subject of the question, Jacobs–Tate syndrome.

'What legal recreational drug exerts some of its effects via an action on the GABA-A receptor?'

Sarah was moving outside her central base of knowledge, but she remembered Thomas once saying something about alcohol affecting the GABA-A receptor and gave this as her answer.

'What are the typical effects of this drug on CNS function?'

'Alcohol is a CNS depressant,' answered Sarah, employing the tactic of beginning with a broad answer. 'It impairs co-ordination, reaction times, judgement and reduces inhibitions.' This aspect of her answer did not require any specialist medical knowledge.

'Through actions on which part of the brain in particular are the effects of this drug on higher function mediated?'

Sarah nearly wrote cerebellum, but then read the question properly and noted the word 'higher'. She recalled some functional neuroanatomy and opted for 'frontal lobes'.

Jacobs–Tate syndrome was no nearer to making any sense to her, but now that Sarah had recovered from her initial dismay on skimming the paper, she could see that she had a fighting chance of squeezing marks out of it.

'How does Cyanococcobacillus jacobstateii survive phagocytosis?'

Sarah's immediate thoughts on reading this would not have borne repetition in polite company. Her next thoughts were that with this question her source of marks from the Jacobs–Tate syndrome SAQ had dried up. However, the mention of surviving phagocytosis triggered a memory from the time she had been rescued from one of Professor Roland Pauls' interminable rambles by one of the Professor's registrars.

Working on the basis that writing nothing would score nothing, Sarah chose to use her knowledge of TB.

'The organism is able to prevent fusion of the lysosome with the phagosome,' she offered.

'What form of inflammatory response might result as a consequence?'

Continuing with her TB analogy, Sarah wrote 'Granulomatous'.

'Name one other sexually transmitted disease that can generate this type of inflammatory response.'

The more important thing for Sarah here was not that she scored another mark by answering syphilis, but that she inferred from the question that *Cyanococcobacillus jacobstateii* was transmitted sexually.

'What characteristic, but non-specific clinical feature does this produce in the vaginal wall or testes of individuals infected with Cyanococcobacillus jacobstateii?'

Thinking again of TB, Sarah associated granulomas with fibrosis and the ability to produce a mass effect, so she answered 'mass or nodule'.

'With what other diagnosis may this cause confusion, especially in the male?'

Sarah reasoned that the differential diagnosis of a mass, especially in the testis, had to include a malignant tumour.

'How do colonies of Cyanococcobacillus jacobstateii migrate from the genital tract to home to the olfactory bulb?'

Sarah did not have a clue as to the specifics, but her understanding of parallel concepts in embryology and the function of inflammatory cells suggested to her that *Cyanococcobacillus jacobstateii* possessed cell adhesion molecules which recognized targets that were specific to the olfactory bulb.

'What clinical features can occur in the non-secretory CNS phase of Jacobs–Tate syndrome?'

Until a few minutes ago, Sarah had never heard of Jacobs–Tate syndrome and it was a further revelation to her that the disease had phases. Her first reaction was to give up on the question, but she glanced at her watch and saw that she was on schedule for the paper and so had time to think.

'It's an infection, causes granulomas, presumably fibrosis and is inside somebody's head,' mused Sarah. 'And it likes the olfactory bulb. So these must be the reasonable features in that case.'

Giving the general clinical features of a chronic intracranial space-occupying lesion, Sarah wrote 'headache and seizures'. Focusing on the specific site, she added 'impaired sense of smell'.

'What clinical features are attributable to the two neurotoxins ethano-benzodiazapoid A and ethano-benzodiazapoid B that are produced by Cyanococcobacillus jacobstateii in the secretory CNS phase of Jacobs–Tate syndrome?'

Now Sarah realized the link between the opening parts of the question and Jacobs–Tate syndrome. She recapitulated her earlier answer regarding the effects of alcohol and added in 'drowsiness, increased sleep and anxiolytic effect', to reflect the actions of benzodiazepines.

'Variant strains of Cyanococcobacillus jacobstateii have reduced or absent synthesis of the two benzodiazapoid neurotoxins. Why could this be a disadvantage in the spread of these variant organisms between individuals?'

Sarah read over the answers she had already given, on the basis that everything she knew about Jacobs–Tate syndrome was in them. After a minute, she worked out that as the disease was sexually transmitted, anything that increased sexual activity, or higher risk sexual activity without barrier contraception, would facilitate spread of the organism. As *Cyanococcobacillus jacobstateii* preferentially targeted the frontal lobes with neurotoxins that had actions which looked like they induced a state resembling a degree of drunkenness, variants of the organism which were defective in the synthesis of these neurotoxins would lose the advantages of the effects of the toxins on promoting sexual behaviour. Realizing that the effects of the neurotoxins were concentrated on the frontal lobes by simple anatomical proximity of the focus of bacterial infection, she decided to delete the effects on co-ordination from her answer to the previous question.

Feeling rather pleased with herself for having kept her head and worked through the question, Sarah's concentration was disturbed by the sound of Kelly shouting abuse at one of the invigilators, a mild-mannered gentleman who worked as an office assistant in the medical school registry. Kelly appeared to be under the misapprehension that the poor man was personally responsible for setting the paper. His attempts to calm Kelly down were ineffective and the student became more and more agitated and aggressive. The reaching out of a hand by the man to soothe her was met by Kelly ramming her fountain pen into his neck with a degree of anatomical precision for the carotid artery that might have gathered marks if the subject of the exam had been surface anatomy.

Before Sarah knew what had happened, she and Kelly were sprinting headlong from the examination hall and through the nearby park. Exactly how or why she had come to accompany Kelly on her flight was unknown to Sarah, she was simply aware that one moment she had been sitting in her chair and the next she was several dozen metres away and that it made perfect sense, even though it simultaneously should not.

For a few seconds, the high-pitched, intrusive and irritating noise sounded like an alert of some sort to Sarah, not really like a police siren, but something similar, perhaps a call to arms or battle stations. After a few more seconds, she had woken up sufficiently to realize it was her alarm clock.

Sarah tried to make sense of her bizarre dream while she brushed her teeth. She remained convinced that she had never heard of Jacobs–Tate syndrome by the time she had made breakfast, but was equally persuaded that all the answers she had given in the paper she had imagined were in themselves correct.

An internet search failed to reveal any references to Jacobs–Tate syndrome, *Cyanococcobacillus jacobstateii* or ethano-benzodiazapoids, leaving Sarah to conclude that while it was all the product of her nightmarish fantasy, she had been able to invent a disease merely through a knowledge of some principles of pathology and perhaps more importantly for the rest of her finals, that a knowledge of its pathology had permitted her to make sense of a disease of which she had otherwise never heard.

NORMAL VALUES

Haemoglobin (Hb)	
men	13–18 g/dL
women	11.5–16 g/dL
Mean cell volume (MCV)	76–96 fL
Mean cell haemoglobin (MCH)	25–35 pg
Mean cell haemoglobin concentration (MCHC)	31–36g/dL
Platelets	$150–400 \times 10^9$/L
White cells (WCC)	$4–11 \times 10^9$/L
Neutrophils	40–75%
Lymphocytes	20–45%
Eosinophils	1–6%
ESR (erythrocyte sedimentation rate)	
men	0–15 mm/h
women	0–20 mm/h
International normalized ratio (INR)	0.9–1.1
APTTR (activated partial thromboplastin time ratio)	0.9–1.1
TT (thrombin time)	14–16 s
Fibrin degradation products	<10 mg/mL
Glucose	3.5–5 mmol/L (fasting)
Urea	2.5–6.7 mmol/L
Creatinine	70–170 μmol/L
Na^+	136–145 mmol/L
K^+	3.5–5.0 mmol/L
Ca^{2+} (corrected)	2.1–2.8 mmol/L
pH	7.35–7.45
PaO_2	>10.6 kPa
$PaCO_2$	4.7–6 kPa
HCO_3^-	22–28 mmol/L
Base excess	±2 mmol/L
Bilirubin	3–17 μmol/L
ALT (alanine aminotransferase)	5–35 IU/L
AST (aspartate aminotransferase)	5–35 IU/L
ALP (alkaline phosphatase)	30–150 IU/L
Albumen	35–48 g/L
GGT (gamma glutamyl transferase)	0–50 IU/L
TSH (thyroid stimulating hormone)	0.5 5.0 mU/L
T4 (thyroxine)	64–155 nmol/L
IgG	6–13 g/L
IgA	0.8–3 g/L
IgM	0.4–2.5 g/L

INDEX OF CONDITIONS COVERED IN CASES

This book is designed to encourage you to think and use your knowledge to answer the structured questions; that means that we did not want to tell you the diagnosis for each case in the title. Here is the list of main conditions covered to help you look for a specific topic.

INDEX

Disorders listed in the 'index of conditions covered in cases' on page 201, have been given page references in bold type.